Clinical Observation
in Communication Sciences
and Disorders

Clinical Observation in Communication Sciences and Disorders

Nancy E. Hall, PhD, CCC-SLP

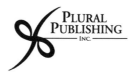

PLURAL
PUBLISHING
INC.

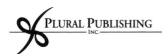

PLURAL PUBLISHING
INC.

5521 Ruffin Road
San Diego, CA 92123

e-mail: info@pluralpublishing.com
Web site: http://www.pluralpublishing.com

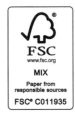

FSC
www.fsc.org
MIX
Paper from
responsible sources
FSC® C011935

Typeset in 10.5/13 ITC Garamond Std by Achorn International
Printed in the United States of America by McNaughton & Gunn

Library of Congress Cataloging-in-Publication Data:

Names: Hall, Nancy E. (Nancy Edna), 1959– author.
Title: Clinical observation in communication sciences and disorders /
    Nancy E. Hall.
Description: San Diego : Plural Publishing, [2019] | Includes bibliographical
    references and index.
Identifiers: LCCN 2017054451| ISBN 9781635500196 (alk. paper) |
    ISBN 1635500192 (alk. paper)
Subjects: | MESH: Communication Disorders—diagnosis | Observation—
    methods | Professional-Patient Relations
Classification: LCC RC423 | NLM WL 340.2 | DDC 616.85/5—dc23
LC record available at https://lccn.loc.gov/2017054451

CONTENTS

SECTION II
Elements of Clinical Observation

PREFACE

Observation is at the heart of any clinical endeavor. It is the integration of knowledge, skill, experience, and expertise within a global perspective as applied to the individual. All that we gain as clinical practitioners factors into the care with which we take to address the needs of our clients or patients—and that process begins, continues, and ends with observation. This text addresses the development of observation skills in communication sciences and disorders (CSD) with the novice clinician or student in mind. It uses a broad approach in considering what is important to learn about observation at the very beginning of a career. The book is not structured around particular speech, language, hearing, or swallowing impairments or what to look for in specific communication disorders. Instead, the focus is on observing the observer, the clinician, and the client/patient. Readers will encounter a great deal of research involving what we bring to the observation process and how our own perspectives can affect what it is we "see" or "hear." We will explore what characteristics to look for in the clinician and the client/patient and how those features impact the therapeutic relationship. A few notes about the text and how it may be best used are in order.

- This book is primarily for undergraduate CSD students who are about to begin or are in the process of obtaining clinical observation hours. Some folks who are already providing clinical services may find it useful as a way of reminding themselves about clinical skills beyond those associated with a diagnosis or therapeutic process.
- Students (particularly undergraduates) may find some of the material and writing a bit challenging. As stated, a fair amount of research is covered in the book. It is included for a number of reasons. First, it is essential that we recognize the value of research in informing our practices. Second, students (perhaps undergraduates especially) need to develop a level of comfort with reading and understanding the literature. All of us can benefit from the practice of reading, synthesizing, and integrating the research into clinical practice. Evidence-based practice requires these skills. Third, much of the research discussed is gleaned from disciplines other than CSD. In part, this is because the CSD literature on observation is somewhat scant, but also because we can learn a great deal from the work of others. And, that brings me to my next point . . .
- The approach in the book is intentionally broad—global, you might say. Observation skills are not unique to CSD professionals, nor to North American professionals!

- Emphasis is given to medicine, nursing, and allied health disciplines, largely because these professions have similar educational and training practices to CSD. Medicine, in particular, has a rich history of explicitly examining observation as an essential skill to be developed and nurtured. Furthermore, these disciplines continue to investigate aspects of training related to interprofessional education and practice with best client/patient outcomes in mind.

- Quite a few concepts, frameworks, and models are discussed in the text. It is not expected that students at the point of clinical observation will learn and retain all of this information. Rather, the goal is to expose students just starting out to aspects of the discipline, such as some of the World Health Organization's efforts, levels of observation, the biopsychosocial model, and the therapeutic alliance. Down the road, students who continue on in CSD will recall being exposed to them and be better able to integrate them into a larger fund of knowledge and skills.

- The text is meant to be supplemental to a class on clinical observation or clinical procedures. Although examples, tables, and figures are included to assist in digesting the material, students are likely to need an instructor or clinical supervisor to help them along the way. A number of exercises are included to assist in identifying and practicing many of the important concepts and skills. It is quite likely that individuals at different stages in their academic and clinical careers will "take away" different points, ideas, and impressions from the text. Therefore, students are encouraged to hang on to the book throughout their developmental process—you may find yourselves referring back to certain concepts as you learn and grow!

- Clinical certification in audiology does not require observation hours. Still, the book addresses clinical observation in CSD as a discipline, discussing concepts, knowledge, and skills that are applicable to both audiology and speech-language pathology professions.

- Many of the exercises contained in the book are designed to be conducted with one of the videos available in the Clinical Video Library. Still, they are written in such a way that they readily can be adapted to other observation experiences.

ACKNOWLEDGMENTS

Thanks to Maggie Pierce, graduate assistant, for her many contributions and for juggling so many tasks, including managing clinical observations, so that I could complete this book. Thank you to the generations of students who have helped me conceptualize the teaching and learning of clinical observation and to the faculty and staff of the CSD department at the University of Maine for their support. Special thanks to Lorriann Mahan, MS, CCC-SLP, who exemplifies what it means to be a master clinician. Most importantly, gratitude is expressed to the clients, patients, and family members for all that they have taught me about observation and life. And lastly, thanks to my son, Sam, for his love and support.

CONTRIBUTORS

Patrick Finn, PhD, CCC-SLP
Professor
Communication Sciences and Special Education
University of Georgia
Athens, Georgia

Marisue Pickering, EdD
Professor Emerita
Communication Sciences and Disorders
University of Maine
Orono, Maine

REVIEWERS

Plural Publishing, Inc., and the author would like to thank the following reviewers for taking the time to provide their valuable feedback during the development process:

Katharine Blaker, MS, CCC-SLP
Clinical Instructor
Department of Speech & Hearing Sciences
University of New Mexico
Albuquerque, New Mexico

Jacqueline Busen, AuD, CCC-A, FAAA
Clinical Assistant Professor
Department of Speech and Hearing Science
Arizona State University
Tempe, Arizona

Barb Cicholski, MA, CCC-SLP
Clinical Assistant Professor
Speech, Language, and Hearing Sciences
Purdue University
West Lafayette, Indiana

Cheryl D. Gunter, PhD, CCC-SLP
Professor and Chairperson
Department of Communication Sciences and Disorders
West Chester University
West Chester, Pennsylvania

Holly S. Kaplan, PhD, CCC-A
Clinical Professor
Communication Sciences & Special Education Department
University of Georgia
Athens, Georgia

Jeanne McMillan, EdD, CCC-SLP
College of Health
Department of Speech Pathology and Audiology
Ball State University
Muncie, Indiana

Emily Patterson, AuD, CCC-A
Clinical Assistant Professor
Department of Speech Pathology and Audiology
Marquette University
Milwaukee, Wisconsin

Deborah Rainer, MS, CCC/SLP
Clinical Coordinator/Senior Lecturer
Department of Communication Sciences and Disorders
Baylor University
Waco, Texas

Gayatri Ram, PhD, CCC-SLP
Assistant Professor
Associate Director of Clinical Education
Pacific University
Forest Grove, Oregon

Bess Sirmon-Taylor, PhD, CCC-SLP
Associate Dean of the UTEP Graduate School
Associate Professor of Speech-Language Pathology
University of Texas at El Paso
El Paso, Texas

Caterina Staltari, MA, CCC-SLP
Director of Clinical Education
Department of Speech-Language Pathology
Duquesne University
Pittsburgh, Pennsylvania

Denise Stats-Caldwell, MA, CCC-SLP
Clinical Associate Professor
Speech and Hearing Science
Arizona State University
Tempe, Arizona

To my father, the original master physician, who walked the talk—reminding me that the provision of quality clinical care requires life-long learning: "That's why they call us practitioners . . . we'll never know it all . . . but we will always be practicing and learning."

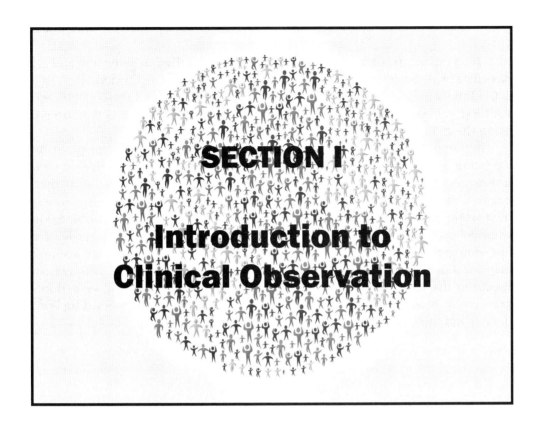

SECTION I
Introduction to Clinical Observation

Observational skills, honed through experience with the literary and visual arts, bring together in a timely manner many of the goals of the medical humanities, providing thematic cohesion through the act of seeing while aiming to advance clinical skills through a unified practice.

—Wellbery and McAteer (2015, p. 1624)

We begin with an introduction to clinical observation. This overview embraces a philosophical orientation in which observation is elevated to a process of clinical practice. We use an historical approach in which we review work conducted on the development and use of keen observational skills in health care disciplines, in particular, medicine. The rationale for looking back within the medical field is, primarily, because that is where the literature leads us. Interestingly, the history of medical education, the instruction and guidance of future physicians, includes a great deal of philosophy. And those in charge of the knowledge and skill development of future physicians have put considerable effort into conceptualizing and carrying out their responsibilities. We would be remiss not to take advantage of their work.

Second, this section scaffolds the pursuit of observation onto a framework for organizing what it is we see, hear, and touch. That organization is grounded in a humanistic approach to understanding communication behavior and its disorders. The reader is introduced to the World Health Organization's (WHO, 2001) International Classification of Functioning, Disability, and Health (ICF) and the biopsychosocial model. We explore how to interpret what it is we observe using these lenses.

Importantly, the reader will want to make note of the author's viewpoint. As a practitioner and an educator, I feel strongly that a broad perspective on clinical matters is of great value. None of us can *know* the experience of another, but all of us can take the time to *appreciate* it. The more we seek to expand our own world views and ways of thinking, the better equipped we will be to do what is best for our clients/patients/students. Whether it is a youngster having just immigrated to my community from Somalia, a 95-year-old veteran seeking help for a hearing loss, a parent with a toddler recently diagnosed with autism spectrum disorder, a young adult recovering from a car accident, or a third-grader who is working on written language, we bring our *best* by devoting both the *art* and the *science* of our profession to each one.

The Art and Science of Clinical Observation

Learning Objectives

- The reader will learn to view clinical observation more broadly than just looking for signs of a communication or swallowing disorder, using models and principles from medical education.
- The reader will learn four levels of observation and eight principles of observation.
- The reader will learn American Speech-Language-Hearing Association's (ASHA's) requirements for clinical observation.
- The reader will learn about humanism in clinical practice.
- The reader will learn about arts-based and visual thinking strategies for enhancing observation skills.

We need to be systematic and rigorous at the same time that we are intuitive and empathetic.

—Berger (1980, p. 356)

Introduction to the Process of Clinical Observation

Clinical observation is more than looking and listening for particular signs or symptoms. It includes more than jotting some notes or transcribing behavior. It is a process, a process that brings together personal beliefs, academic knowledge, and clinical experience with a context that includes the perspectives, values, and needs of clients and patients and their families. Because the process of clinical observation relies on the development of well-honed skills, it must be practiced again and again. And it must be grounded in a sound philosophy supporting clinical practice.

Using Inductive and Deductive Reasoning

Manton (2004) explains that being skilled at observation involves much more than having the knowledge set. When conducting clinical observation, both inductive and deductive reasoning processes, as well as intuition, are involved, and the interaction of these processes with scientific knowledge and past experience goes into describing what is observed, using inference and interpreting multiple components of the clinical picture. The process of inductive reasoning, sometimes thought of as "bottom–up" thinking, involves the bringing together of parts to explain a whole or to support a conclusion (depicted in Figure 1–1). Typically, observations are made through which a pattern may be detected and we develop a tentative hypothesis on the basis of that pattern. We then test our hypothesis within the realm of available theory. In clinical observation, this might be likened to identifying signs or symptoms, collecting data on specific components of communication, and comparing this information to what is understood to be the norm for a particular culture. In contrast, deductive reasoning, or "top–down" logic, applies theoretical knowledge to hypothesis testing, often employing a set of rules or laws (or deductions) to come to a true conclusion. Figure 1–2 presents the process of deductive reasoning.

As an example, with inductive reasoning, one might use the following observations in determining an hypothesis of possible deafness:

a. The child is older than two years.
b. The child has been exposed to appropriate language models in her environment.
c. The child does not respond to her name.
d. The child uses gestures, body language, grunts, and cries to make her needs known.
e. The child enjoys playing interactive games.

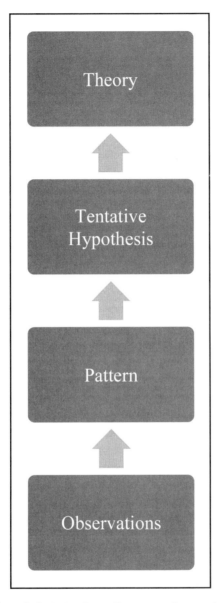

Figure 1–1. Inductive or "bottom–up" reasoning.

In contrast, a deductive process of clinical reasoning, albeit faulty, might look like this:

a. All children with autism spectrum disorders have impairment in social skills.
b. This child has social skills impairment.
c. Therefore, this child must have an autism spectrum disorder.

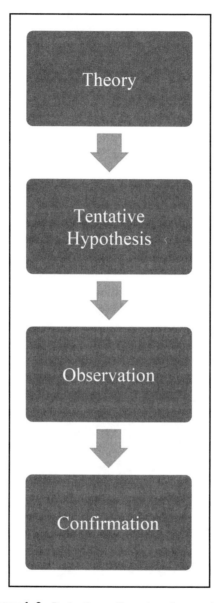

Figure 1–2. Deductive or "top–down" reasoning.

Developing Hypotheses

Using these processes in making observations allows the skilled practitioner to develop multiple hypotheses regarding the clinical picture into which she or he can integrate scientific knowledge and clinical experience. Hypothesis testing and using multiple methods of reasoning embody the "science" of communication sciences and disorders (CSD). In using the steps of the scientific method, we employ a standard practice that allows us to carefully scrutinize our evidence in the context of what is to be expected and in comparison to appropriate normative information.

Scientific Evidence and Intuition

Intuition, on the other hand, is not rooted in the science of the discipline. It is largely an instinctive, rather than consciously reasoned, process of assigning meaning. When we use intuition as a guide, we rely on a "gut feeling" or a sense of how something "seems" to be. An example of the use of intuition might look like this: We observe a child who uses echolalia and can see that its use does not facilitate communication. Thus, we intuit something is awry with the child's communication on the basis of the presence of the echolalia. The intuitive process may be quite familiar, and some clinicians may rely on it in decision making; however, intuition is not the same as clinical judgment. The use of clinical judgment is dependent on the development of expertise, a component of evidence-based practice. As a discipline in which best practices are expected to be evidence-based, CSD does not condone the use of intuition in clinical work. Therefore, it is important that future clinicians learn to recognize the ways in which we might approach clinical decision making, and work to hone those skills that align with best practice philosophies. In Chapter 3, we explore the various ways in which we might explain beliefs, behavior, and feelings that are developed over the course of personal and professional growth and how those "Ways of Knowing" fit into observing clinical practice.

Thus far, I have attempted to introduce the reader to the art and science of CSD. Often, it is the integration of these components that can be shortchanged, circumvented, or left out altogether, allowing the clinician to miss the mark on diagnosis and/or treatment. Although there may be truth to the adage that experienced clinicians know what they see and those with less experience may see only what they know, there is no guarantee that only with experience does one develop expert skill at observation along the way to becoming a master clinician. Certainly, experience is of considerable value, yet those clinicians new to the field may have a certain advantage in that they will be fresh from having their skills scrutinized, critiqued, and sharply honed. Thus, whether you are a clinician with many years under your belt, a student just beginning the journey, or a newly minted practitioner, your skill at observation is likely to be the most important tool in your clinical repertoire.

There is good reason why the education and training of communication disorders professionals include attention to both knowledge and skills. Practitioners in the disciplines of audiology and speech-language pathology are expected to amass a substantial amount of critical knowledge regarding human communication and swallowing processes, potential impairments, etiological factors, signs, and symptoms, as well as elements of diagnosis and intervention. And, of course, the treatment of communication impairments is not reliant solely on that knowledge. Rather, clinicians must develop and practice the myriad clinical skills essential to quality clinical care. One of the first steps toward obtaining and mastering skills in clinical fields is to recognize the role of observation, to learn what is involved in successful observation, and to practice critical observation skills. To better understand the centrality of observation to clinical practice, an historical journey is in order.

An Historical Perspective

Perspectives on the value of observation in clinical practice have been around for a long time. In 1889, Charcot spoke about observation as essential to the development of clinical competence in the physician (as cited in Huth & Murray, 2006). Clinical observation is a fundamental skill, one that must be cultivated through training and experience, and continually practiced. A look at the history of observation in medicine reveals pedagogical and practical support for providing direct, guided training in observation skills. To get the most out of observation, one must approach the task with a foundation of what observation is, how important it is, and a theoretical perspective on observation. So, what might these principles of observation look like?

Clinical Observation in Medicine

In 2008, Boudreau, Cassell, and Fuks (2008) outlined principles of observation in their description of a course on clinical observation designed for first-year medical students. To begin with, the principles are grounded in Berger's (1980) hierarchy of observation. Berger, a physician, articulated four "levels" of observation, with each serving an essential function in the process of providing quality medical care. The levels, presented in Table 1–1, can be seen as providing a fundamental method for approaching a clinical case. Each of these levels has associated goals. At the first level of observation (Level 1), which Berger identified as gathering "clinical material," the clinician attends to information and data with a goal of determining the presence of impairment or differential diagnosis. The second level (Level 2) is aimed at personal description of the patient, something that can be characterized as objective or subjective. Understanding the differences between these two types of description is key to quality clinical care and will be addressed further in Chapter 2 when we detail a framework for observation.

Table 1–1. Berger's Levels of Observation

Level 1: "Clinical material" of history, physical, and laboratory results

Level 2: Description of personal characteristics of appearance and behavior

Level 3: Description of interactions

Level 4: Insight into the clinician's own feelings and behaviors

Source: Adapted from Berger (1980).

The focus of Level 3, description of interactions, is at the heart of our work in the discipline of CSD; after all, we are in the business of communication, which is the bedrock of interaction. Berger (1980), in his work as a pediatrician, comments as to the value of observing what *is* (italics added) working in addition to what might not be working well, ". . . to be able to characterize the child and family in terms of their strengths and weaknesses, their healthy dynamics as well as possibly maladaptive ones. . . . recognizing families that are functioning *well* (italics in original) is also of great value" (p. 357). Finally, the fourth level of observation may be the most difficult one for clinicians to embrace. It includes the actualization of one's own needs, concerns, values, biases, feelings, etc. It is the recognition that we, as human communicators ourselves, are important components of the observation context. At this level, we must ask ourselves, "What is my experience with this circumstance?" "How do I know what it is I am observing?" "Do I have my own preconceived ideas regarding what I am observing?" While continually debated, the process of this type of self-actualization has been a part of the training and development of such professionals as clinical psychologists (Macran & Shapiro, 1998; Malikiosi-Loizos, 2013) and psychiatrists (Habl, Mintz, & Bailey, 2010); yet, it is not routinely explored for the majority of health care practitioners.

The notion of "humanism" as essential to functioning as a well-rounded, expert clinician has been debated in the medical education field for generations (e.g., Katz & Khoshbin, 2014; Novak, Epstein, & Paulsen, 1999). In a testament to the importance placed on the "human side" of medicine, the Association of American Medical Colleges (AAMC) recently revised the Medical College Admission Test (MCAT) to include assessment of psychological, sociocultural, communication, and critical thinking skills in addition to the traditional basic science assessment.[1] In clarifying the changes to the MCAT, and recommendations provided to medical colleges, Dr. Darrell G. Kirch, president and chief executive officer of the AAMC, pointed to patient perspectives on health care. As indicated in an interview with *New York Times* reporter Elizabeth Rosenthal in 2012, Dr. Kirch stressed the desire of many patients to be more connected with their doctors (e.g., "the public had great confidence in doctors' knowledge but much less in their bedside manner"[2]).

Thus, we see that those in the business of educating and training physicians have come to recognize that assuring quality health care goes beyond making sure the doctor is smart and well grounded in the science of medicine. The move

---

[1] See https://aamc-orange.global.ssl.fastly.net/production/media/filer_public/7f/bc/7fbce904 -eff1-425d-a6b1-b29a770f0176/updatesummarycoursemappingtoolv2.pdf for an explanation of recent changes to the MCAT.

[2] http://www.nytimes.com/2012/04/15/education/edlife/pre-meds-new-priorities-heart -and-soul-and-social-science.html?rref=collection%2Fbyline%2Felisabeth-rosenthal&action =click&contentCollection=undefined&region=stream&module=stream_unit&version=search &contentPlacement=95&pgtype=collection.

toward expecting incoming medical students to have an educational background that includes the humanities and stressing the importance of heeding patient concerns regarding their health care providers is evidence that the foundation underlying the practice of clinical work must include the pillars of both art and science. These principles and aspects of patient/client satisfaction and quality characteristics of clinicians are further addressed in Chapters 4 and 5.

Having determined the levels of observation, we return to the principles outlined by Boudreau et al. (2008). These authors, physicians involved with the education of medical students, recognized that clinical observation was something that needed to be taught directly, and the processes of teaching and learning clinical observation need to be supported with theoretical and pedagogical foundations. Eight "core principles" were developed by Boudreau et al. as a means of capturing the whole of the clinical observation experience and to provide guidance to others arranging observation experiences for new students. These eight principles are listed in Table 1–2, and described below.

Boudreau et al. (2008) describe observation as having both "sensory perceptive" and "cognitive" aspects (Principle 1), meaning that not only does the clinician observe through looking at the patient or client but also, much of the observer's information or impressions may be perceptive in nature and are naturally informed by the experiences and knowledge the observer brings to the observation experience. I would further add that the sensory perceptive component is much broader than simply looking or seeing. As clinicians, we rely on a multitude of senses (seeing, hearing, and touching) and incorporate sensory impressions with emotions, as well as knowledge. Identifying elements through observation naturally incorporates judgment of what we observe and often leads to inference. Inference involves drawing some type of conclusion on the basis of evidence and reasoning, which may or may not be sound. Boudreau et al. cautions the clinical observer to be mindful of making rushed inferences based on less than valid or reliable evidence.

Table 1–2. Principles of Observation

(1) Observation has a sensory perceptive and a cognitive component.

(2) Observation is distinct from inference.

(3) Observation is made concrete through description.

(4) Observation occurs on different levels.

(5) Observation is goal oriented.

(6) Observation occurs over time.

(7) Observation is subject to powerful cultural determinants.

(8) Observation carries ethical obligations.

Source: Adapted from Boudreau, Cassells, and Fuks (2008).

Other principles outlined by Boudreau et al. (2008) involve structural components, such as having a specific goal outlined, observing on multiple different levels, using concrete description, and making observations over time. Such aspects of the observational process may seem straightforward or self-evident; however, they require planning, just as do other elements involved in clinical observation. Without planning and providing for the opportunity to observe certain aspects of a patient's or client's life or behavior, a less informed picture will emerge. For example, standard practice in stuttering assessment requires the client provide samples of speech from a variety of settings while interacting with a number of different people. Making such a request addresses the principles of observation on multiple levels (Principle 4 in Table 1–2), having goals for the observation (Principle 5 in Table 1–2), and ensuring that observation takes place over time (Principle 6 in Table 1–2). Thus, the clinician is afforded the opportunity to observe client behavior and social factors in relation to speaking behavior and the client's knowledge and feelings about stuttering.

Ultimately, observation must be consistent with ethical clinical practice (Principle 8 in Table 1–2). Clinicians are responsible for how they record, interpret, and use their observations. The observer is reminded that ethical conduct is expected. This includes how one conducts oneself on-site, the manner in which observations are recorded and discussed, and most importantly, the attitudes and actions with which one regards clients and patients. Your conduct has implications for the supervising clinician as well. Each and every client/patient observed is or has been served by a clinician holding national certification from ASHA. That clinician is bound by ASHA's Code of Ethics and ultimately responsible for the care of those you observe. It is in the best interest of all that you be familiar with the code (http://www.asha.org/Code-of-Ethics/).

It is vital that bias and cultural considerations be recognized as potentially influencing the ways in which observations are construed (Principle 7 in Table 1–2). Past research demonstrates that there is a relationship between ethical practice and a connection to the humanities (Coles, 1979). In his description of the challenges that quality physicians face when balancing scientific knowledge and technical advances with the "human" side of medical care, Coles (1979) submits that the farther removed the physician is from using clinical observation and spending time interacting with the patient, the more likely errors of ethical conduct are to occur. Katz and Khoshbin (2014) argue these outcomes are a result of ". . . over reliance on exotic tests and therapies, professional burnout, and a public that recognizes the value of the scientific advances while simultaneously distrusting that the profession has patients' best interests at heart" (p. 331). Although all of us are greatly influenced by culture, experience, and knowledge, it behooves us as clinicians to recognize the roles that these factors may play in our processes of deduction, induction, hypothesis development, and the drawing of inferences (Principle 2 in Table 1–2). We will be discussing these elements further in Section II when we look at our "ways of knowing" and how we use past experiences and personal biases when approaching the observation process.

Clinical Observation in CSD

The history of clinical observation in CSD is brief and without detail. The ASHA Council for Clinical Certification in Speech-Language Pathology and Audiology sets forth the national certification standards for clinical practice (Certificate of Clinical Competence; CCC). These standards are organized around knowledge (typically academic) and skills (typically practical), and they specify both the coursework and clinical practice experiences required. Among the clinical hours needed for the CCC in speech-language pathology (SLP) are 25 hours of supervised clinical observation (the standards for the CCC in Audiology do not require observation hours at all). Beyond specifying the number of observation hours required, the CCC-SLP standards contain the following language regarding implementation of the observation hours standard:

> Guided observation hours generally precede direct contact with clients/patients. The observation and direct client/patient contact hours must be within the ASHA Scope of Practice in Speech-Language Pathology and must be under the supervision of a qualified professional who holds current ASHA certification in the appropriate practice area. Such supervision may occur simultaneously with the student's observation or afterwards through review and approval of written reports or summaries submitted by the student. Students may use video recordings of client services for observation purposes (2014 Standards and Implementation Procedures for the Certificate of Clinical Competence in Speech-Language Pathology, http://www.asha.org).

Beyond this brief description, academic programs and students are provided little in the way of theoretical or pedagogical rationale for why the attainment of 25 hours of clinical observation is important to the development of a skilled clinician. Even the implementation language is unclear as to when observation hours are expected to be obtained. In a recent survey of academic CSD programs, I found considerable variability in how observation hours are delivered to CSD students and in the ways in which these students are expected to report on their observations (Hall, 2016). In particular, more than a third of the programs reported providing no direct training or instruction in clinical observation, and just a little more than 50% indicated explicit objectives associated with observation experiences. These findings reveal what appears to be a fragmented approach to helping students gain experience through clinical observation. Yet, there is value in obtaining observational experience, particularly if it is guided by experts in the field—a concept we will explore throughout this text. An example of a model for observation used in CSD comes from Emerick and Hatten (1974). In it, the authors outline five components central to organizing clinical observation. These are defined in Table 1–3, with a broader description and an exercise in applying them offered in Exercise 1–4.

Table 1–3. Model of Observation

Element	Description
Focus	The first step in observation is to focus on a very descriptive level so that the examiner can present the actual behaviors the client exhibited rather than generalizations regarding the meaning of those actions. In order to underscore the importance of focusing attention in the observational task, we often ask students to observe some single aspect of behavior in a therapy session and report on that one characteristic.
Depth	The depth of the observation is determined to a large degree by circumstance, but the diagnostician must find ways to observe the client interact with many different people and stimuli. The diagnostician cannot expect to gain a great deal of information from fleeting observations; she or he must be willing to spend the time and energy necessary to observe a significant amount of the behavior.
Description	In the early stages, the diagnostician must train herself or himself to describe behavior in writing as objectively, explicitly, and completely as possible. During these first attempts to communicate the findings of the observation, the clinician must withstand the temptation to jump to conclusions. She or he must stick to what she or he observes and what she or he can describe.
Interpretation	Once all pertinent behaviors have been described, it is incumbent upon the observer to make *interpretations*. At this point, the observer makes inferences regarding the meaning of behaviors; she or he attempts to generalize and classify behaviors and draw conclusions as to the meaning of what she or he observed.
Implications	The observer is expected to explain the *implications* of the observed behavior—the impact the behavior has on communication, how significant that impact is, how malleable the behavior is, etc. Implications can include statements about potential causes or etiologies and prognosis. The observations should be written in such a way as to assist in determining treatment options.

Source: Adapted from Emerick and Hatten (1974).

It seems that delivering guided observation experiences that expose beginning CSD students to the breadth and depth of the discipline, along with providing them a framework and a set of principles to help structure their observations and self-growth would go a long way toward shaping a new generation of master clinicians. In the following sections, I discuss the value of clinical observation as it relates to the development of a whole clinician, that is, a master clinician as embodied by the "compassionate scientist" portrayed by Goldberg in his 1997 book on clinical skills. Further, I present a paradigm for guided observation as developed in the field of medical education, and how it may be applied to clinical observation in communication sciences and disorders.

The Importance of Clinical Observation in Developing the Master Clinician

According to Goldberg (1997), compassionate scientists are those "who intensely care for the well-being of their clients, and endeavor to meet their needs in the most effective, scientific manner" (p. 313). This concept has long been espoused in the field of clinical psychology (e.g., Raimy, 1950), where practitioners have been expected to develop research knowledge and skills in addition to clinical knowledge and skills. Of note is what has been termed the "Local Clinical Science Model," a process of "disciplined inquiry, critical thinking, imagination, rigor, skepticism, and openness to change in the face of evidence," which is applied in the practice setting through the development of hypotheses and the collection of evidence (through interactions with the client/patient, testing, interviewing, etc.) to support or refute one of more hypotheses (Stricker, 2002, p. 1278). The exploration of what makes a quality practitioner often traces the same path as scientific advances in clinical practice. As is the case in health care, the ability to gain more and more precise diagnostic information through sophisticated tests using state-of-the-art machinery has made the clinician's job all the more technical. All clinical practitioners face the same pressures—to align practices with third-party billing procedures, to become proficient at using electronic data systems, to maintain high caseloads in order to offset the expenses of additional materials, tests, etc. And research suggests that these forces often conspire to reduce practitioners' time, job satisfaction, patient satisfaction and trust, and importantly, client/patient outcomes (Friedberg et al., 2013). In fact, many have bemoaned the impact these factors have had on clinical observation expertise, suggesting the reliance on test results that are believed to be irrefutable has given practitioners false confidence in their skills and provided a way to avoid true provider-to-patient contact (Fred, 2014; Grais, 2014).

In the fields of audiology and speech-language pathology, we have enjoyed relative immunity from many of these influences, thus far. In general, practitioners in the CSD discipline express high job satisfaction,[3] and audiologists and speech-language pathologists have been ranked by Careercast as top-rated jobs for a number of years.[4] With this in mind, I would suggest that we are in the enviable position of taking advantage of efforts by other health care disciplines to address some of the shortcomings previously identified. In specific, a great deal has been said about the failings of health care in client/patient satisfaction. Over and over, the message has been that consumers of health care find the system daunting, and in many cases, dehumanizing. What they want is a practitioner who has the knowledge, expertise, and experience to inspire confidence; at the same time, they expect their health care provider to recognize them as fellow human

---

[3] http://leader.pubs.asha.org/article.aspx?articleid=2292188
[4] http://www.careercast.com/jobs-rated/jobs-rated-2014-ranking-200-jobs-best-worst; http://www.careercast.com/jobs-rated/jobs-rated-report-2015-ranking-top-200-jobs

beings. Time spent on the skills of observation will help with the development of those characteristics that clients/patients most want in their providers (see Chapters 4 and 5 for more on practitioner and client/patient qualities).

What does all of this have to do with clinical observation in CSD, you might ask? I would argue that when stripped of the tests, diagnostic materials, and procedures, and all the attendant pressures of the bottom line, the practitioner is left with experience, the cognitive processes of the scientific method, fundamental skills of observation, and humanism. These components are essential to quality clinical care, beginning with observing and experiencing the human condition. That is to say, the provision of quality clinical care includes as much art and humanity as it does science.[5]

So, how does a cramped CSD curriculum prepare students in arts and humanities as well as in basic science, the course of human communication and swallowing (both normal and disordered), observation, evidence-based practice, clinical procedures, and interprofessional practice? I believe we have a lot to learn from how other disciplines have tackled this dilemma. In particular, prominent medical education programs have taken pains to examine the underpinnings of the "compassionate scientist" in providing essential humanistic experiences to medical trainees and have developed a model of incorporating arts and humanities into core activities designed to assist students in developing a broader, more humanistic perspective. In the following section, I explore some of the work that has gone into these efforts.

A Paradigm for Guided Observation

Much of the recent work on clinical observation in medicine has involved the direct teaching of skills fundamental to observation through the implementation of arts-based activities (e.g., Braverman, 2011; Dolev, Friedlaender, & Braverman, 2001; Katz & Khoshbin, 2014; Klugman, Peel, & Beckman-Mendez, 2011; Miller, Grohe, Khoshbin, & Katz, 2013; Perry, Maffulli, Wilson & Morrissey, 2011). For example, both Harvard and Yale medical schools have implemented coursework involving the exploration of visual art to teach aspiring medical practitioners to take care in observing—recognizing both the complexities of observing what might be considered unfamiliar (i.e., visual art pieces as compared to standard medical biological, anatomical, and physiological features) and how the observer brings a wealth of information, beliefs, and biases to the observational context.

In their 2011 review of the research on medical education using arts-based teaching paradigms, Perry et al. describe the procedures as aimed at ". . . foster[ing] understanding of the patient's perspective and . . . enhancing communication skills. . . ." (p. 141). By exposing medical students to or requiring them to

---

[5] Many thanks to Susan K. Riley, MS, CCC-SLP, for the numerous enlightening discussions of CSD and the liberal arts.

participate in literature, drama, art, and music, medical educators aim to expand a future doctor's perspectives on the human condition. And although Perry et al. found that such experiences appear to positively impact students' attitudes about their patients and can be translated into greater empathy and understanding for the patient as a person, at the time of the study, the authors concluded that there exists limited evidence for the effectiveness of arts-based experiences in the development of specific observation skills.

The effectiveness of arts-based training in observation has been tested using a collaborative model with both physician-to-be and nursing students (Klugman et al., 2011). The researchers expanded on the more common model of art-based education by bringing together medical and nursing students to work on "visual thinking strategies" in their process of observing and describing works of art. Visual thinking strategies, a process developed to help foster empathic understanding of others' experiences of art, are methods used by many disciplines to teach collaboration among teams (such as health care providers), improve observational descriptions (as used by police detectives for crime scenes), and increase thinking skills in school children (Housen, http://www.vtshome.org). Using a pretest and posttest design, Klugman et al. (2011) examined the effects of visual thinking training on medical and nursing students' impressions of art, their level of comfort with ambiguity depicted in works of art or patient images, and the assessment of their own communication skills. Statistically significant differences were found when comparing measurement of the previously mentioned skills before engaging in discussions of art and patient images led by museum staff and those measured after the discussions. The authors interpreted these findings as suggesting that more time spent looking at, discussing, or contemplating images translates into improved observations. In learning to take the time to carefully examine an image (or a patient or client), the researchers speculated that medical and nursing students afforded themselves enhanced data collection and greater possibility to partner with the patient (or client), leading to improved health care. The findings of this study not only provide support for the use of arts-based observation training and visual thinking strategies but also show that students developed greater comfort with ambiguity and reflected positively on the opportunity for interprofessional collaboration. It has been suggested that tolerance of ambiguity is associated with greater openness to patients' input,[6] and much has been said about the importance of interprofessional collaboration in the provision of quality health care (e.g., Johnson, Prelock, & Apel, 2016). We will revisit the notion of "tolerance of ambiguity" when discussing clinician characteristics in Chapter 4.

So, what might be a paradigm for guided clinical observation? I propose that, rather than view the observation requirement as a hurdle to jump, we regard it as an opportunity to provide future clinicians with expanded ways of thinking, keen observation skills, and practice in integrating the art and science

---

[6]Academic Medicine Blog: http://academicmedicineblog.org/what-does-tolerance-for-ambi guity-look-like/

of the CSD discipline. The medical education literature shows us that students develop enhanced observation techniques and greater confidence in clinical observation skills through direct teaching using arts-based activities. The growth of a skilled clinical observer can be facilitated through pairing description of what is being observed (e.g., a painting) with engaging in collaborative activities of meaning-making (i.e., Interprofessional Education activities) and bridging these experiences to actual clinical cases (Miller et al., 2013; Naghshineh et al., 2008). In my institution, I have partnered with faculty from the Department of Art to present new ways of "observing" to my class on clinical observation. Another possibility to help students with these skills might be to bring together students from different disciplines (e.g., pre-med, nursing, and allied health) to engage in a workshop using arts-based activities for practicing observation, verbal description, and the sharing of perspectives.

The following chapters present arts- and science-based concepts and exercises consistent with the principles of observation outlined earlier. Students can expect to be challenged to consider both objective and subjective points of view, reflect on their own strengths and weaknesses relative to the fundamentals of clinical practice, tolerate ambiguity, use visual thinking strategies, and work collaboratively to build mutual meaning and understandings. We use a four-element model that includes exploring clinical observation (and the clinical process) from the perspectives of the observer, the clinician, the client, and the client–clinician relationship.

Before we explore the four elements, I present a framework for observation that includes basic structural components such as how to organize an observation, set goals, and record information. Whether the observation experience is related to the requirements of a course or just because you are interested in learning more about clinical work in CSD, one should always have at least one goal in mind. What we bring to the observation will influence what it is we get out of the experience. How we conduct ourselves will affect the types of opportunities provided us, and the manner in which we collect information can impact how much we learn.

Finally, the reader is introduced to the WHO ICF and the biopsychosocial model. These models are designed with the client/patient at the center, to consider all of the facets of being human before determining diagnosis or disease. Engel (1977), a physician and prominent proponent of the biopsychosocial model, provides a quote from art historian E. H. Gombrich, who well describes the notion of uniting science *and* art in clinical practice:

> For why should we perpetuate that false opposition between science and art which gives to art what is murky, instinctive and by definition inaccessible to rational discussion? It finds no warrant in either psychology or history. Many scientists have testified to the role which creative dreams have played in their work, dreams that were hammered into rational theories by hard and inspired work; many artists, on the other hand use the power of intellect with a lucidity and concentration that rivals that of scientific power. (p. 222)

Chapter Summary

This chapter introduces a new perspective on clinical observation. More than simply looking for evidence of a communication disorder, the experience of observation involves recognition of the many components of clinical practice. Further, students of CSD can begin immediately the work of honing observation skills by learning what it means to "look and see" and "hear and listen" and applying both "art" and "science" to the process. An historical perspective is presented as a way of "stepping back" and capturing a larger view of the process of observation and where it fits in the realm of clinical practice. As beginning clinicians, it is important to remember that what one "sees" can be organized according to context, behavior, and that which is not spoken, as well as be interpreted through our own experiential lenses. We can assist ourselves in developing keen observation skills by practicing observation. In the following observations and exercises, we will apply some of this chapter's principles to observation and begin that all-important practice.

Chapter Observations and Exercises

Below are exercises designed to help you develop a broader, open-minded approach to observation. Some of them are directly related to clinical observation, and some are designed to give you practice at framing observation in different ways. The exercises linked to clinical observation are written with "Jon" (in our Clinical Video Library) in mind; however, you can conduct the exercises with any clinical observation.

Exercise 1–1

Observation is not just "looking." And when we "look," are we "seeing" what we want to see, or what we are familiar with? Take a look at Figure 1–3. What do you see? Ask a classmate to describe what she or he sees? What about this image strikes you? What kinds of experiences or feelings does the image evoke? In viewing this particular piece, could you image different reactions to it depending on a person's perspective? How could this exercise help you in developing clinical observation skills? Consider visiting a local art museum, theater, or concert to continue practicing art observation. Bring along a friend or classmate, or

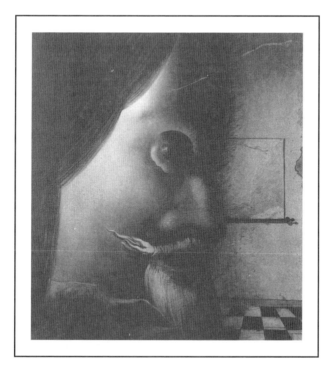

Figure 1–3. The Image Disappears (Dali, 1938). *Source:* https://www.salvador-dali.org/en/artwork/the-collection/140/the-image-disappears

better yet, ask your instructor to arrange an art gallery visit with an art instructor or artist to facilitate your observation experience.

Exercise 1–2

1. After viewing the first 5 to 10 minutes of the Jon video, develop hypotheses for the following:
   a. Why the client is seeking therapy
   b. Possible goals for the session
2. Outline an *inductive* reasoning process to support your hypotheses for (a) and (b) in Item 1 above. Your process should look something like what is pictured in Figure 1–1.
3. Outline a *deductive* reasoning process to support your hypotheses for (a) and (b) above. Your process should look something like what is pictured in Figure 1–2.

Exercise 1–3

Along with clinical observation, this exercise uses a variety of activities to explore the principles of observation we covered in this chapter. As a first step, review the principles presented in Table 1–2.

A. Explain the difference between description and inference. Why is it important to understand that observation is distinct from inference?

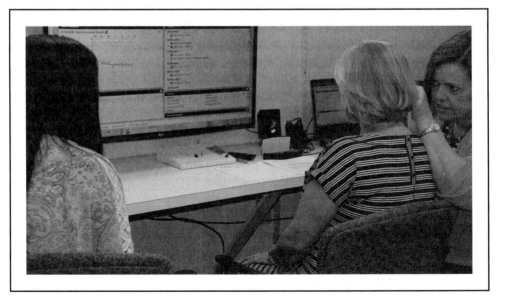

Figure 1–4. Accompanies Exercise 1–3.

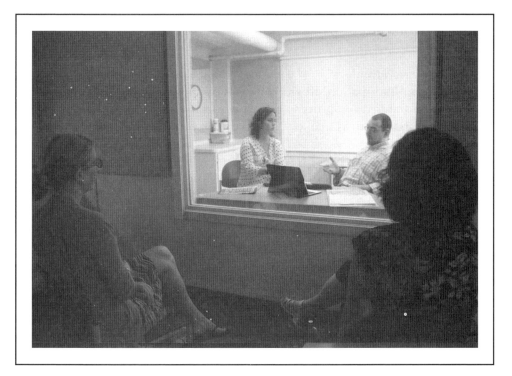

Figure 1–5. Accompanies Exercise 1–3.

B. View Figures 1–4 and 1–5. Note your observations and describe them. Share with your classmates your descriptions. How are they the same/different from others'? What did you learn from the discussion of the different descriptions?

C. Spend another 5 to 10 minutes observing Jon. Jot down any notes regarding observations you make—don't be concerned with the accuracy of your notes or how well they are written. These notes can be about the client, the clinician, what you see, what you hear, reactions you have, questions that come up, ideas you might like to follow-up on, what you wish you knew about the client, the clinician . . . pretty much anything. Once you have finished taking notes, identify which ones reflect

   a. sensory perceptive or cognitive processes.

   b. description versus inference.

   c. different levels of observation.

Exercise 1–4

Use the model described in Table 1–3 to structure your next observation and report. While developed with diagnosis and evaluation in mind, the five elements it contains are well suited to organizing clinical observation: *focus*, *depth*, *description*, *interpretation*, and *implications*. For this exercise, we will attend to the first three components of the model. *Please follow the outline below (each step has an in-depth description) to write your report.*

1. Prior to observation:
   a. Based on information provided to you by the clinician, identify three aspects of the therapy process, which will constitute your *focus*.
   b. Identify how you will collect your data for your *focus*.

Note: The first step is to choose a *focus*; you are going to want to focus on a very descriptive level and you should choose at least three aspects of the session that you can observe and describe. This can be a client behavior, a clinician behavior, a teaching strategy, and so on. Simply choose the aspects of the session you will observe and decide how you will collect the data.

2. Following the observation:
   a. *Describe* clearly and concisely the observations you made related to your *focus*.

Note: Using the data you gathered, you will describe in detail, using concise terms, all of your observations related to your focus. Do not make a judgment or write a personal reaction to what you observe. Describe what you saw based on your data.

3. If you were to have the opportunity to observe the client in *depth*, what different settings or contexts would you choose for the observations? Give your reasons for choosing these.

Note: Imagine that you have the opportunity to observe the client in depth. Think about what you have been observing and the questions that arise and think about another context or setting that might help you learn more about what you have been observing.

Exercise EXTRA!

Many stories exist that tell the tales of families and individuals experiencing disability, handicap, or impairment. They can be found in film, books, blogs, websites, podcasts, etc. Some of these chronicle the experiences families and persons with disabilities have interacting with health care providers, educators, and/or rehabilitation specialists. Read/view/listen to one of these stories (I have included a list in the Appendix) and reflect on how the relationships between the practitioners/clinicians/teachers/etc. and the individuals and their families are described. What do you see as key to the success or failure of these relationships? How could you incorporate what you have learned from this experience into your own approach to the profession of audiology or speech-language pathology?

A Process, a Framework, and a Model for Clinical Observation

Chapter Outline

Learning Objectives

- The reader will learn the value of and practice setting observation goals.
- The reader will learn the difference between objective and subjective writing.
- The reader will practice describing what is being observed by writing about the environment, people, and treatment plan.
- The reader will learn the International Classification of Functioning, Disability, and Health (ICF) Framework and be able to identify components of it as they relate to observation.
- The reader will learn the philosophy behind a biopsychosocial model to clinical practice.

Students must first learn what it is to see with an open mind. Next, they must practice the act of describing what they see to help them develop the communication skills needed to articulate what is ailing and what improvements are feasible. Finally, they must develop the ability to craft this speech with others—sometimes called public narrative—which can lead to interventions that have positive impacts on themselves, their colleagues, and patients.

—Wellbery and McAteer (2015, p. 1624)

Developing a framework or structure for observing the clinical process helps you focus and allows you to gather information to establish a foundation and understanding of what it is you are observing. At the outset, a specific goal or goals for the observation can enhance the experience. In many ways, the actual goal set may not be as important as the fact that you have identified something to focus on. So, where to begin with setting goals? Well, for some, the goals may be determined by an instructor or supervisor, and for others, they may be self-determined. The types of goals you set likely depend on how much experience you have. For the novice observer, an appropriate goal may be to learn how speech-language pathologists (SLPs) and audiologists conduct business on a daily basis. A more advanced observer may focus on the behaviors of the clinician, for example, how the clinician uses questions or open-ended comments to elicit information from the client. A valuable exercise for any observer is to practice setting goals that can be applied to a variety of observation experiences. As we move along in this chapter, we will develop several goals to guide our observation experiences.

Setting Goals

For students just learning about the discipline of communication sciences and disorders (CSD) and the provision of therapeutic services, a primary observation task may be to "survey" a variety of settings, clients/patients, and circumstances. Thus, a first goal might include observing or job shadowing SLPs and audiologists in several settings, such as hospitals, rehabilitation settings, schools, and/or clinics. In visiting these facilities and observing how the professionals conduct their business, not only will you learn about what a typical day might look like, you will also gain valuable experience in conducting yourself professionally.

Once you have had the chance to look at the "bigger picture" of clinical practice through visitations at various settings, you will be ready to tackle more specific goal setting. The remainder of this chapter presents components of a framework for organizing observation and focuses on developing objective, rather than subjective descriptions in detailing our observations. Following that, we will practice describing the setting, the people involved, and the therapeutic plan through the activities presented at the end of the chapter. In later chapters, we will focus less on extrinsic factors and more on clinical behaviors and interactions.

Learning to Write Objectively

Recently, a great deal has been said about the role of bias or subjectivity in how we go about our daily lives. A quick Internet search using the terms *bias in everyday life* reveals millions of hits, with the top items coming from news sources or sites in which one can learn more about signs of bias or test oneself for possible bias. For example, lifehack.org published a blog on how 20 different cognitive biases can impact our decision making.[1] These might include a tendency to give greater weight to information we've received more recently or if it is more salient to us. Also, we are more likely to accept and rely on information that is consistent with our own experiences. Clinically, these possible biases have the potential to lead us in making decisions that may not be in the best interest of our clients or patients. Sometimes, biases, even implicit ones we may not be aware of, can have far-reaching implications. Take, for example, the notion of a "confirmation bias," which is the use of certain processes or procedures that will naturally confirm our hypotheses. A story I like to tell my students comes close to illustrating confirmation bias. In my second year as a practicing SLP, I worked as a research assistant on a large nationally funded research project involving the assessment of a significant number of preschool children with developmental disorders. In the early months on the job, before I was to begin seeing participants in the project, my supervisor asked me to conduct a few diagnostic assessments under her guidance. In one such case, after administering several diagnostic tests and collecting a spontaneous language sample on a young boy, I came away puzzled about what was going on with the child. I shared the test results and impressions with my supervisor and expressed my bewilderment as to the youngster's diagnosis. She examined the findings carefully, then looked at me and said, "Nancy, not all of the children you see will have a problem. This child's speech and language is within normal limits." There I was—I had assumed the youngster would present a speech and/or language impairment simply because he has been brought to me for assessment. Had I continued to scrutinize every little piece of data obtained from that boy, chances are I would have eventually found something to confirm my hypothesis that a speech and/or language impairment was present.

None of us can escape holding biases. In fact, most research indicates that biases or stereotypes are very difficult to eliminate (e.g., Burgess, van Ryn, Dovidio, & Saha, 2007). Still, that same research suggests that biases can be controlled to a degree (Blaire, 2002). One of the most effective ways of doing so is to help clinicians remember their clients or patients as individuals, real people, rather than as their diagnoses. We can work to develop a clinical style in which we

---

[1] http://www.lifehack.org/340263/aware-these-cognitive-biases-and-youll-much-more-successful

Table 2–1. Objective Versus Subjective Writing

Objective	Subjective
The mother was observed to smile each time her son pointed to a picture.	The mother was happy her son was pointing to pictures.
After approximately 10 minutes, the patient said he was tired and closed the book.	The patient lasted only about 10 minutes before giving up.
The child produced 10 out of 15 utterances correctly using the target vocabulary.	The child seems to know the vocabulary because she said most of them correctly.
The session included three activities, during which each of the three children participated by responding to the clinician's model.	The children in the group liked the activities because they all took turns.
The patient coughed repeatedly after each attempt to swallow thin liquids.	The patient didn't like to swallow thin liquids and kept coughing.

continually ask ourselves about the nature of the information we are using, on what evidence we are basing observations, and if there may be alternative perspectives that could inform our clinical practice. This type of approach to clinical work can be enhanced through frequently practicing the use of objective description. Throughout your career as an audiologist or SLP, you will be expected to use objective language to inform others about your clinical practice.

The difference between subjective language and objective language is that on which a statement is based. In writing observations, we must be careful to include factual, observable information. What can be seen? What can be heard? Observations that are carefully described and include factual information can be considered objective. In contrast, subjective is often based on feelings, hunches, or perceptions. In cases with subjective language, what is reported may not be observable. Consider the examples provided in Table 2–1. Review these, then turn to the end of the chapter and complete Exercise 2–2 to practice recognizing and differentiating subjective from objective description.

Describing the Context

Along with setting goals, your observation should be centered on describing the context. Imagine you are explaining to another student, a clinician, or a clinical supervisor what you observed. Before getting to aspects of the client's speech, language, or hearing impairment, or how the clinician conducted therapy or the session, you must set the stage. Primarily, this involves describing the environment and the people included in the session. Of importance is that you do so objectively. This is not the time for judgment or interpretation.

In accordance with Berger's (1980) levels of observation, understanding the context is included in Level 1. At this level, the observer is gathering information, collecting data as a way of facilitating insight to the individual separate from any diagnosis. Berger's explanation of this level involves activity that typically would be done prior to seeing the individual (such as reviewing any previous test results) or while examining the person (such as conducting an oral mechanism examination). Nevertheless, the observer who is not participating in the session still has much information to collect that can be useful in understanding the client/patient and clinical circumstances. In some cases, the clinician being observed may provide background information, or the observer may have the opportunity to speak with a family member about the client/patient. In these cases, it is important for the observer to make note of such material and include a statement as to its source. Again, objectivity is paramount.

Observing the Environment

First, one must identify the setting. Is the observation taking place live, via some type of recording, through an observation medium, or directly? It is important to describe these factors because how one approaches the observation, whether or not the observer is present within the session, and the type of environment will impact the interpretation or meaning given to the information collected. As an example, an observer who is sitting within a classroom in which an SLP is conducting group therapy may have the opportunity to directly interact with the children being served, whereas an observer who is viewing a recording of a session will have no opportunity to observe behavior directly. In some cases, the presence of the observer may serve to motivate or intimidate clients or patients such that the behavior observed and the subsequent collection of information or data may not reflect what happens in a typical session. Further, if the observer is unable to determine the exact nature of the setting (e.g., is only able to see or hear a small portion of the environs), then she or he must clearly note only what is observable. Table 2–2 includes suggested facets of the environment to observe and record. Exercise 2–3A provides the opportunity to practice describing the environment.

Table 2–2. Observing the Environment

Setting	Type of space, size of space, decor, etc.
Seating	Type of seating (or not), arrangement of seating, etc.
Structures present (e.g., table, window, etc.)	
Materials	Types of materials, placement of materials
Sounds	Sounds internal to or external to room

Table 2–3. Observing the People

---

(1) Who is present? (Client(s)? Clinician? Family? Approximate ages? Etc.)

(2) What are the relationships among the players?

(3) What role(s) do the people play? (Observer? Communicator? Facilitator? Etc.)

Observing the People

Level 2 of Berger's hierarchy encompasses the person—"personal characteristics of appearance and behavior." For our observation purposes, we must include a description of all of the people involved. This means identifying who is present in the session, their relationship with each other, and the role each plays (see Table 2–3). At this point, it can be more difficult to be objective in our descriptions as we naturally want to make appraisals of people and how they impact the person with the communication disorder. If we keep in mind that we are only attempting to set the stage, describe the context of what it is we are observing, we will have an easier time using objective language to describe the various players. It is also important to remember that, at this point, we are simply interested in describing the people, not the behavior. Turn to the exercises at the end of the chapter. Exercise 2–3B affords you practice at developing your own descriptions from a spontaneous observation.

Observing the Communication Behavior

Having gained experience with setting goals, and describing the setting and people, we can turn our attention to aspects of the communication disorder and components of the therapeutic process. These facets are consistent with Berger's Levels 1 and 2 as we are still identifying and recording information about the setting and the individual. Most likely, those of you completing clinical observation experiences have yet to be exposed to all that CSD involves. I suspect most of you have been busy studying the processes of normal human communication and swallowing, in order to better understand how things might go wrong. Thus, when observing for behaviors consistent with different types of communication or swallowing disorders, we want to be extra careful that we not let our own assumptions, beliefs, and experiences shade how we take in what it is we are observing. Whereas the description of a client's hearing, speech, and language necessitates a certain judgment, it is important to consider that description can be done without identifying impairment. Again, a good rule of thumb is to imagine that another student or clinician (or even another student or professional from a different discipline) will be reading your description. Your job, then, is to illustrate or depict the speech, language, and/or hearing without projecting your own beliefs or diagnosis into the description. A considerable amount of your time will be spent observing and describing communication behavior. The process of doing so requires practice, feedback, and more practice. Several exercises along these lines are presented at the end of this chapter and throughout the book. Many of these can be used multiple times as you conduct observations in different settings, with different clients/patients and different clinicians.

The reader is referred to the Hambrecht and Rice (2011) text on clinical observation as a good resource for organizing information and describing behaviors in CSD.

Observing the Session

Lastly, we want to gain information about the goals and objectives of the session we are observing. In order to do so, we need to know something about treatment plans or the structure of diagnostic sessions. For each client or patient, the SLP develops an assessment or treatment plan, which will include specific goals, objectives, activities, and outcomes. Specified in the treatment plan are the changes in speech and language we expect to effect (see Table 2–4 for SLP treatment example). These elements depend on the nature of the treatment, who the client/patient is, and the overall expectations for therapy. For example, a client who has recently returned home from a lengthy stay in a rehabilitation center because of a traumatic brain injury may have multiple goals focusing on many aspects of communication, such as ways to communicate daily needs, retrieving basic vocabulary, or regulating verbal output. In audiology, for a client/patient whose primary concern is ringing in the ears, the types of diagnostic procedures, interview questions, and counseling behaviors will differ from those used with an individual who recently received a cochlear implant. For the observer, if possible, it will be

Table 2–4. Observing the Treatment Plan

The treatment plan includes the following:

(1) Goals:	Broad changes in communication behavior expected over time. For example: "Meg will increase her ability to be understood from 50% to 80% of the time to an unfamiliar listener within a known context."
(2) Objectives:	Steps developed to assist client in making progress toward overall goals. For example: "When provided with at least six pictured minimal pairs, Meg will verbally reduce the process of fronting and produce the /k/ and /g/ sounds at the word level spontaneously in 90% of attempts."
	Performance—What the learner is supposed to do.
	Condition—The conditions under which the learner will perform.
	Criterion—The level at which the learner must perform to have achieved the objective.

helpful to have an understanding of the clinician's goals for the session. In some cases, as an observer, you may not have enough information to adequately detail the treatment plan. If that is true, you will need to rely on basic description of the types of activities and materials used, as well as the behavior exhibited by both the clinician and the client. Numerous resources exist for assisting students in determining the structure of a typical treatment or assessment session in either SLP or audiology. The reader is referred to the American Speech-Language-Hearing Association's (ASHA's) practice portal for information and disorder-specific guidelines (http://www.asha.org/practice-portal/), and the exercises at the end of this chapter. We will address how to observe both the clinician and the client in later chapters in Section II.

The final exercises in this chapter provide opportunities for you to practice identifying goals, objectives, activities, and outcomes for both SLP and audiology sessions. Once you have completed these exercises, you will have gained valuable experience with the first two levels of Berger's hierarchy of observation. Furthermore, you will have practiced several of the principles of observation outlined by Boudreau, et al. (2008). You will have conducted observations that were goal oriented, used both sensory and cognitive processes, occurred on different levels, and were made concrete through description. Reflect on the skills you have developed thus far. Are there skills that still need practice? Are you ready to advance to observing interactions (Berger's Level 3) and consider your own feelings and behaviors (Berger's Level 4) in relation to observation and clinical practice?

A Global Framework and Model

This text asserts the use of two additional frameworks and a conceptual model: The World Health Organization's (WHO's; 2001, 2007) International Classification of Functioning, Disability, and Health and its Child and Youth frameworks (ICF and ICF-CY) and the biopsychosocial model approach to client/patient care (Engel, 1977, 1997). A brief description of both is provided here, and each is elaborated on in additional chapters.

The ICF Framework

The WHO promotes itself as the "Global Guardian of Public Health" (2016). It is a global organization whose mission is to promote health for all people. Among its many efforts are the eradication of disease; promotion of the health of women, babies, and children; rebuilding of health care systems in areas of strife; and addressing mental illness. Over decades, the WHO has developed different systems for classifying life function and disability, which include the ICF and ICF-CY. These are designed to provide frameworks, including a uniform language and coding scheme, from which practitioners in different disciplines across the world can work. They are different from the *International Statistical Classification of Diseases and Related Health Problems* (Version 10; ICD-10; WHO, 1990), which is a system for classifying disease and health problems as a means for tracking public health trends, as well as for cataloguing diagnoses within a practice setting. We will be using the ICF and ICF-CY in this text to help us view communication disorders more broadly. These frameworks include two domains: a health domain, and a health-related domain. Within these domains, information is described from the perspective of the body, the individual, and society within the components of the body (systems and structures), function (activity and participation), and contextual factors (environmental and personal). The ICF and ICF-CY also frame these components as related to disability: activity limitations, participation restrictions, and environmental influences. Keep in mind that "Activity" refers to that which the individual performs (e.g., a task or activity), and "Participation" refers to the individual's performance within society (e.g., "involvement in a life situation"; WHO, 2001, p. 10). Table 2–5 shows a list of the concepts of the ICF Activity and Participation as summarized by Whiteneck (as cited in O'Halloran & Larkins, 2008). Accordingly, the SLP is expected to address both activity and participation. Within the scopes of practice for audiology and speech-language pathology, ASHA has adopted the ICF frameworks for best practice, stating that they can be used in describing various responsibilities of practitioners and the investigation and rehabilitation of communication disorders (ASHA, 2004, 2016b). An illustration of the components of the ICF and ICF-CY is provided in Figure 2–1 and definitions of ICF terms are provided in Table 2–6.

Table 2–5. ICF Concepts of Activity and Participation

Activity	Participation
Individual level	Societal level
Performed alone	Performed with others
Simple	Complex
Related to impairment	Related to quality of life
Less environment dependent	More environment dependent
Medical model of disability	Social model of disability
Focus of rehabilitation	Focus of consumers
Assessed in hospital	Assessed in community
Clinician assessment	Self or proxy report
Not always possible	Always theoretically possible
Task	Social role

Source: Adapted from O'Halloran and Larkins (2008).

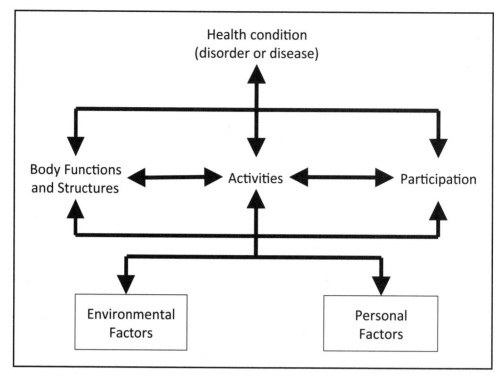

Figure 2-1. The ICF framework. Reprinted with permission from the World Health Organization. (2007). *International Classification of Functioning, Disability and Health: Children and Youth Version: ICF-CY.* Geneva, Switzerland: WHO Press.

Table 2-6. ICF Definition of Terms

Definitions

In the context of health:

Body functions are the physiological functions of the body systems (including psychological functions).

Body structures are anatomical parts of the body, such as organs, limbs, and their components.

Impairments are problems in body function or structure such as a significant deviation or loss.

Activity is the execution of a task or action by an individual.

Participation is involvement in a life situation.

Activity limitations are difficulties a person may have in executing activities.

Participation limitations are problems a person may experience in involvement in life situations.

Environmental factors make up the physical, social, and attitudinal environment in which people live and conduct their lives.

Source: Adapted from World Health Organization (2001).

The Biopsychosocial Model

The biopsychosocial model is a relationship-focused approach (Engel, 1977, 1997). As proposed by Engel, it includes several key elements:

1. The patient (or client) as a "whole," a person whose fundamental nature is at once biological, psychological, and social;
2. A triadic process of observation, introspection, and dialogue through which the patient's (client's) subjective experiences become scientific data;
3. A clinical interview in which the patient's (client's) narrative is allowed to unfold without interruptions and with minimal prompting or interrogation;
4. A practitioner–patient (client) relationship that fosters shared and complementary communication and responsibilities;
5. A mutual understanding of the patient's (client's) narrative that ensures inclusion of his or her perceptions and experiences in the assessment and diagnostic process;
6. Patient (client) engagement in the treatment process and plans that are intended to alleviate or resolve perceived illness or disability; and
7. Systems theory rather than reductionism as the approach to analyzing and understanding health and illness.

In particular, Engel (1977) contends that the traditional biomedical model has no room in it for considering the individual's experience of illness, disease, or impairment. And yet, it is the subjective experience of the patient/client, both from an internal systems and an external systems perspective, that can be as influential as the objective evidence from diagnostic measures in determining the course of treatment.

The beauty of applying the biopsychosocial model to audiology and speech-language pathology is the emphasis it places on communication and relationship building. Notably, observation is identified as a key component of this person-centered approach to providing health care—"participant observation." Participant observation, in this case, means the practitioner is a keen observer while actively participating in the relationship. We will explore the elements of observation using these models when considering the observer, the clinician, the client, and the relationship between the client/patient and the clinician.

Chapter Summary

In this chapter, we review a framework for structuring clinical observations, taking into account features of the session we might be observing. The importance of setting goals for clinical observation is emphasized, along with recognizing various components of the session, such as the environment, people, and therapy plan. Presented is the WHO framework for examining health classification, life functioning, and disability, along with the biopsychosocial model, both important mechanisms for helping us understand the dynamics of providing clinical services. Use these to help you begin organizing communication disorders and their treatment. The exercises at the end of this chapter are designed to give you practice with key skills, such as setting goals, learning to write objectively, and describing what it is you are observing.

Chapter Observations and Exercises

Exercise 2–1: Goal Setting

Goal: I want to learn more about the profession of Audiology or Speech-Language Pathology. Identify three different employment settings in which you would like to observe. Develop a plan for observing in those settings. Your plan should include appropriate contact information, a description of the reasons for observing, what you hope to accomplish, and if you have an assignment associated with the observation. Be sure you have a list of questions you will want answered *before* you go to conduct the observation. Your list should include the following:

- Does the facility have a specific protocol for student observers? (For example, many work settings require observers to provide immunization records and contact information of the class instructor and expect observers to attend an orientation.)
- Who is the primary contact for student observers?
- Where is the facility located? Where can I park? Do I need a parking pass? Is there bus, train/subway, or shuttle service?
- Do you have a dress code?
- Will I need an ID?
- How much time am I expected to commit to observing?
- Will I have the opportunity to speak with the audiologist/SLP before, during, or after the observation?

Once you arrive and have met up with the clinician or clinicians you will be observing, be sure you understand the expectations. Keep in mind that the clinician's primary responsibility is the client's or patient's welfare. Confidentiality, the protection of client or patient information, is of utmost concern. Many employment settings will expect observers to sign forms promising confidentiality. It is always good to remind ourselves that the people we encounter have granted permission to be observed for educational purposes and they deserve our gratitude and respect. Basic questions to ask when preparing to observe include the following:

- Is there a secure place for me to store my belongings?
- Where is the restroom located?
- Will I be expected to observe from a particular space or be allowed in the room?
- Is it appropriate for me to interact with the client or patient and their family?
- Will there be a time and place appropriate for asking questions?
- What is the best way to thank the client/patient?

When your observation is complete, be sure to thank the clinician for her or his time and for helping you learn more about the profession. If you are expected to provide a written summary or other assignment to your instructor, it would be respectful to ask the clinician if she or he would like to see it before you turn it in. Also, follow up your observation with a handwritten note thanking the clinician and the facility for their generosity in providing you the opportunity to observe.

A good rule of thumb for all on-site observations is as follows: Conduct yourself professionally in appearance and manner. Remember to be polite and respectful—there is a good chance you may encounter that clinician again in the future, as you advance in the profession.

Employment setting possibilities may include the following:

Audiology	Speech-Language Pathology
Hospitals	Schools
Rehabilitation facilities	Hospitals
Nursing homes/Long-term care	Rehabilitation facilities
Schools	Clinics
Private/Group practice	Private/Group practice
Federal/State government	Skilled nursing facilities
Uniformed services	Federal/State government
Clinics	Corporate SLP
Public health	Public health
Hearing conservation	Uniformed SERVICES

Exercise 2–2: Differentiating Between Objective and Subjective

Read the following statements and determine why they might be considered subjective. How might you re-write them to be more objective?

1. "The boy didn't like the activity, so he crawled under the table."
2. "The client never used the strategy correctly because she just wasn't trying hard enough."
3. "The clinician worried the family didn't like her and that's why they were always late to therapy."
4. "The client never took care of his hearing aids and was always bringing them in for repair."
5. "After a short time, the patient began yelling and cursing at the clinician for no reason."

Exercise 2–3: Describing What We See

A. Describing the Environment
After observing for 5 to 10 minutes, record your observations of the environment (setting, sounds, materials, seating, other, etc.). Keep in mind that you want

to use objective descriptive language that "paints a picture" of the environment. Compare your observations with those of a classmate and identify any similarities and differences.

B. Observing the People

After observing for 5 to 10 minutes, record your observations of the people (who is involved, what is their role, how does each person contribute, and others). Keep in mind that you want to use objective descriptive language that identifies the people and their involvement in the session. Compare your observations with those of a classmate and identify any similarities and differences.

Exercise 2–4: Observing Communication Behavior

Taking notes on communication behavior can be challenging. Following the model presented in the last chapter's exercises, you will want to identify a focus. Perhaps you want to focus on certain aspects of hearing, speech, swallowing, or language. There are a myriad of aspects of communication that can be observed. For starters, keep it simple. With a classmate, determine two or three foci that you each will attend to for a specified period of time. Be sure your goals are appropriate. In other words, it might not make sense to observe a client's articulation skills, when the individual is an adult in therapy for voice concerns, or perhaps the client is a toddler with delayed language, you would not expect to observe much in the way of complex syntax.

Once you have decided on your goals, take careful notes. When you compare your notes with those of your classmate's, how consistent are you with each other? Pay particular attention to the objectivity of the notes and comments you discuss. Be sure to challenge both yourself and your partner to support the observations with evidence and facts.

Exercise 2–5: Observing the Treatment Plan

For this activity, we use the small group session of our clinical video labeled DP and HR. The goals for the segment you will be observing include the following:

- Correct production of bound morphemes (e.g., plural /s/, possessive /s/, regular third-person tense markers, past tense markers, etc.)
- Turn taking
- Narrative skill development

Take notes as to the following:

- What activities did the clinician use to achieve the goals?
- Did the clinician use a particular sequence of activities?
- Why do you suppose she chose the activities she did?

- How successful was she in achieving the goals?
- If you were to modify the session, how might you do things differently?

Exercise 2–6: The ICF Framework

Reproduce the ICF framework. Conduct an observation with the framework in mind. Make notes as to how environmental, health, or personal factors might impact how the client/patient functions in daily life. Identify a specific example from the observation in which the communication impairment is related to body structure/function, activities, and/or participation.

Exercise 2–7: The Biopsychosocial Model

Return to the video of Jon (or select another video in which the client/patient is being interviewed about the communication impairment and therapy). For each of the seven points listed for the biopsychosocial model, identify evidence from the video that speaks to the point or represents an aspect of the model that the clinician will want to consider.

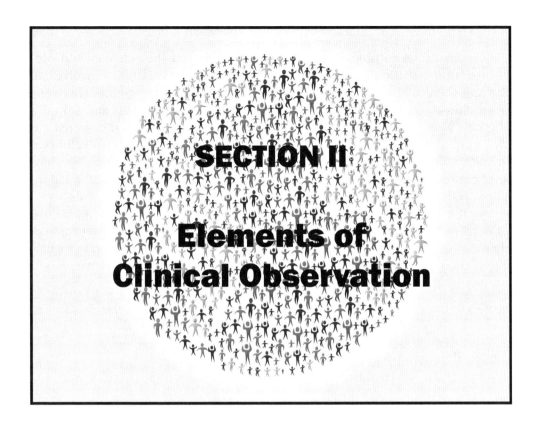

SECTION II
Elements of Clinical Observation

While observing holistically and discovering what catches your attention can be appropriate, 25 hours of unfocused observation may not be making the most of this valuable learning opportunity.

—Hambrecht and Rice (2011, p. xi)

Presented in the introductory chapter is a philosophical approach to clinical observation, grounded in the belief that our ability to make sense of clinical information through observation and data collection can be our most important clinical skill. In the second chapter, we discussed a framework for observation, the importance of having a plan for structuring clinical observation and the basics of the World Health Organization's International Classification of Functioning, Disability, and Health and the biopsychosocial model. This section describes specific elements on which to focus while conducting clinical observation: yourself as an observer (Chapter 3), the clinician and the client/patient (Chapter 4), and the client/patient–clinician relationship (Chapter 5). In addition to having a framework and a plan for carrying out clinical observation, we must understand what we bring to the observation process, what a clinician brings, and how that clinician's perspective, attitude, experience, and so on, play into the success of the therapeutic process. Also, work in clinical practice is not limited to that which the clinician does to prepare for the session, carry out the activities and procedures of the session, and evaluate the session's success but also involves all that the client or patient does to make changes to hearing, speech, language, or swallowing. Certainly, the client/patient brings a host of beliefs and attitudes about services, which will be revealed in her or his behaviors and responses to direction by the clinician. We also examine how the client/patient and clinician interact, focusing on the relationship, something Berger identifies as his third level of observation. He reminds the reader that all interactions and all relationships are important. As an example, he describes how teaching students about neonatal assessment can help them develop an appreciation for the interactive capacities of newborns. At the end of each chapter are a number of exercises designed to explore the elements through different lenses, connected to particular observation experiences.

Element 1:
The Observer

Chapter Outline

Learning Objectives

- The reader will learn about and practice self-reflection and critical thinking as they pertain to clinical observation.

- The reader will identify different ways of knowing.
- The reader will learn about cultural sensitivity and look for elements of this in clinical practice through observations.
- The reader will learn about the value of professional identity and the role communication plays in forming a sense of professionalism.

An aspiring speech-language pathologist is constantly searching for a way to do better and to learn more. The aspiration of clinicians may be contagious in that such aspirations may help clients believe that they can indeed improve.

—Threats (2010, p. 87)

Introduction to the Observer

Here, we start with the observer—you. Berger (1980) makes a point of identifying the clinician as an essential "level" in his hierarchy. He refers to the fourth level as ". . . the most difficult to develop, and potentially the most important to physicians and families alike. It consists of insight into the physician's own feelings and behavior" (Berger, 1980, p. 357). As an observer, using Berger's hierarchy, you must consider yourself a developing clinician, one who brings a unique set of experiences, values, and beliefs to clinical observation. Many of us were first attracted to the field because of the prospect of helping. We may identify ourselves as "helpers" or people who care about other people, interested in "people work" and begin our professional path with first seeing our compassion as pivotal (on our way to becoming the "compassionate scientist"). And this professional journey starts with recognizing who we are, beginning with the practice of self-reflection, identifying how we know what we know, learning to think critically, working toward cultural sensitivity, and cultivating a professional identity.

Self-Reflection

When one conducts a Google web search for "self-reflection," the following definition appears: "meditation or serious thought about one's character, actions, and motives."[1] Self-identity is described as "the recognition of one's poten-

---

[1] https://www.google.com/search?newwindow=1&safe=active&q=self-reflection&oq=self -reflection&gs_l=serp.3..0l10.1395939.1398376.0.1398699.15.12.0.2.2.0.147.1138.6j5.11.0....0 ...1c.1.64.serp..2.13.1146...0i67k1j0i131i67k1j0i131k1.UwjYOG9ExKI

Table 3-1. Exploring Self-Identity

(1) List at least five "qualities" of your self-identity.	
(2) Do you see those features as key to you achieving your goal of becoming an audiologist or speech-language pathologist?	(2a) If so, how? (2b) If not, why not? How might you work to transform them to be more in line with such a goal?
(3) Or, perhaps, having spent time thinking about your "qualities" and "potential," you have discovered another possible path for your future?	

tial and qualities as an individual, especially in relation to social context."[2] The meanings expressed in these definitions are appealing because they both focus on a person; her or his substantive qualities (i.e., "character") *and* behavior (i.e., "serious thought," "motivations," and "potential"). Rather than simply identifying oneself as a student or a clinician, using these descriptions, we can depict ourselves by being mindful of our strengths and weaknesses and how those can be modified to show our potential. With this type of orientation, how might you characterize your self-identity? Take a moment and respond to the questions in Table 3–1.

The point of the activity in Table 3–1 is to facilitate the exploration of oneself as a potential clinician and begin the development of self-reflective skills. The processes involved in treating hearing, speech, language, and swallowing disorders are all about change. To help facilitate change in others, one needs to know something about the process of change in oneself, starting with self-reflection. Borrowing from the academic medicine literature, the exploration of a professional identity is a concept aimed at the education of humanistic physicians, which begins with developing skill at self-reflection (Wald et al., 2015). The push toward assisting students in gaining skill at self-reflection stems from a belief that engaging in an "active construction process" directed at building a professional identity will eventually lead to a clinician who provides better quality care and aids in the advancement of a practitioner who brings the "whole person to whole person care" (Wald et al., 2015, pp. 753 and 758). In nursing, Bulman, Lathlean, and Gobbi (2012) liken reflection to the concept of "critical being," as proposed by Barnett (1997). That is, one engaged in growing into a critical being (or acquiring reflection skills) is advancing ". . . the development of critical thinking . . . the critical development of oneself and the commitment

---

[2] https://www.google.com/search?newwindow=1&safe=active&q=self+identity&oq=self+identi&gs_l=serp.1.0.0l10.375125.379144.0.381960.11.8.0.3.3.0.133.755.3j4.7.0....0...1c.1.64.serp..1.10.778...0i67k1j0i131i67k1j0i131k1.W7jHo6HhRv8

to take action in the world" (Bulman et al., 2012, p. e12). The abilities to engage in critical thinking and implement reflection as related to professional skill development do not simply appear, they must be taught, worked on, and cultivated. In communication sciences and disorders (CSD), the development of critical thinking skills (and companion reflection skills) has been identified as essential for the advancement of speech, language, and hearing professionals and quality clinical decision making, as well as foundational to successful interprofessional practice (IPP; Finn, Brundage, & DiLollo, 2016). Thus, in acquiring self-reflection skills, one is engaging in processes of critical thinking that will directly impact the provision of clinical services. We will return to the discussion of critical thinking skills following an exploration of reflection and how we might acquire the ability to reflect on ourselves and practice.

So, what exactly is reflection and how do we acquire the skills necessary to be a mindful, reflective clinician and advance a professional identity for ourselves? If we refer to the biopsychosocial framework, we recognize that Engel's (1997) "introspection" is another word for reflection. Both students and clinicians benefit from reflective learning and reflective practice. To be a *reflective learner*, one engages in examining experiences from multiple perspectives and uses those perspectives to gain insight that ultimately alters understanding and subsequent action. A *reflective practitioner*, on the other hand, is focused on studying context, action, and outcomes to advance one's self and one's practice. As a student participating in the observation process, you are using reflective learning skills, while preparing yourself to be a reflective practitioner. Jacobs (2016) refers to "authentic reflection . . . [as] . . . not only providing rationales for our actions, but also constantly exploring and examining ourselves and our own growth . . . [it is] action oriented . . . [and] an active process of discovering oneself" (pp. 62–63). More than that, reflection must have identifiable outcomes, as indicated in Jacob's (2016) summary of the nursing literature. These are listed in Table 3–2, and we will return to these in our reflective practice exercises.

One must have a certain capacity for reflection, defined by some as the metacognitive skills and emotional awareness that allow one to use critical thinking in problem-solving and clinical practice (Hill, Davidson, & Theodoros, 2012; Wald

Table 3–2. Reflective Practice Outcomes

Develop coping strategies
Enhance interprofessional communication
Increase students' understanding of nursing practice
Promote the expression of feelings
Make sense of personal emotional practice challenges
Help nursing students to know themselves

Source: Adapted from Jacobs (2016).

et al., 2015). The process used in reflective practice includes specific types of reasoning. According to Mamede and Schmidt (2004), to reflect on one's practice, one must employ "thinking" and "affective" strategies. Cognitive approaches (i.e., "thinking" strategies) include both inductive and deductive reasoning and hypothesis generation and testing. As a student engaging in clinical observation, you will find yourself using cognitive, or thinking, strategies to help you make sense of what it is you are observing. Imagine yourself observing a speech-language pathologist (SLP) providing support to students in a fifth grade classroom. First, you might *think* about what would be expected of fifth graders in terms of communication skills, drawing on what you know about typical speech, language, and learning. Second, you may observe that the SLP is working with a small group of students while they are completing a science project on plant parts and their functions. Thinking through the reasons why an SLP might be involved in the classroom, with a group of students, would lead you to develop some *hypotheses*, such as the following: The SLP is assisting one of the group members with vocabulary development or peer interaction skills, or perhaps, the teacher has requested that the SLP work with different groups in the classroom to facilitate group participation skills. With such hypotheses, you will then want to determine how to best collect evidence to support one or more of them.

The reflective practitioner, however, cannot be successful using only the cognitive strategies but must be open to reflection on feelings or emotion ("affective" strategies) and engage in metacognitive reasoning. That is, a reflective process entails being able to identify the procedures one uses and their effectiveness and determine how well client/patient needs and well-being are being addressed and to have a certain tolerance for ambiguity or uncertainty while assessing one's own beliefs and assumptions throughout the thinking process (Mamede & Schmidt, 2004). As outlined by Hill et al. (2012), "Self appraisal leads to increased insight which leads to enhanced thinking and reasoning" (p. 414). Moreover, enhanced thinking and reasoning are tied to the use of clinical reasoning. We will consider these concepts further in the section below on critical thinking.

Clarke (2014) evaluated the ways in which both undergraduate students and teachers in nursing conceptualize reflective practice involving focus groups. Posed to the groups were interview questions around the definition of reflection, how it is taught, the skills necessary for a reflective practitioner, and ways they might change how reflection is taught and learned. As a result of careful data analysis, in combination with findings from other investigations, Clarke identifies 11 skills that she regards as central to being successful in using reflection. Notably, a majority of the "ingredients" Clarke identifies are affective rather than cognitive. For example, empathy, mindfulness, and appropriate attitudinal characteristics are included in her list. Certainly, academic skill and knowledge also are key components to being a reflective practitioner. As Clarke points out, it is critical that the clinician possess current knowledge or have the ability to obtain it and use strategies to make connections to theoretical information from the clinical domain; that is, "bridge the theory–practice gap" (p. 1224). Along with the cognitive processes, practitioners must have attitudinal and affective characteristics that allow for open, honest, and courageous communication with herself or himself. In order to make such a process useful, the clinician must be mindful and self-aware, recognizing that reflection is about self-growth and is an ongoing part of clinical practice. There is no end point. Clarke makes a point of reminding the reader that reflective practice is not exclusive to nursing and can be useful across many health care disciplines. In clinical observation, this might take the form of not only developing hypotheses about what it is we observe but also recognizing and recording our own reactions—asking ourselves, "How am I feeling about what is transpiring?" "Do I have a personal experience that allows me to see the clinical interaction from different perspectives?" "How do my personal experiences inform my cognitive understanding?" "What theories of speech and language development help me better understand what I am observing?"

How we acquire skill with reflection is not readily determined. A systematic review by Mann, Gordon, and MacLeod (2009) shows that the best circumstances for developing reflection include, among others, support (academic and emotional), expression of opinion, authentic context ("real world" practice), and group discussion. They further point out that reflection is best promoted within learning activities in which students are expected to engage in the creation of meaning related to their reflections. For example, Sobral (2000) finds that medical students' learning experiences are enhanced when greater effort is put into reflection activities. Further, it has been suggested that the presence of a "reflective stance" (i.e., a mindset of using reflection to facilitate learning) may be tied to greater capacity for reflection and its use in diagnostic situations (Sobral, 2005). Sobral (2005) also argues that reflection can be related to a student's sense of responsibility for her or his learning and ability to self-regulate learning. These findings have implications for CSD students, as they begin their academic route to practitioner. It is my contention that practice at reflection prior to engaging in clinical work will aid the student in gaining an understanding of her or his learning style, "reflective stance," and a sense of self as a future clinician. In the United States, the most authentic contexts are not always available to students in audiology and speech-language pathology until they are in graduate school. That is not to say that undergraduate students in CSD are not in a position to begin developing skill in reflection. That is why this text incorporates reflection into the observational experience, something we will explore in the exercises at the end of the chapter.

So, what is known about CSD students' reflective skills? The empirical investigation of the use of reflection by CSD students appears to be limited to a small number of studies (e.g., Baxter & Gray, 2001; Epstein, 2008; Higgs & McAllister, 2007; Hill et al., 2012; Horton, Bing, Bunning, & Pring, 2004; Schaub-de Jong & van der Schans, 2010; Schaub-de Jong, Schönrock-Adema, Dekker, Verkerk, & Cohen-Schotanus, 2011). In their review of the works involving the examination of reflective skills in the field of speech-language pathology, Caty, Kinsella, and Doyle (2015) identify key issues related to how we understand reflective practice. They note that there is little consensus on terminology, identifying eight different terms (reflection, reflective practice, reflective learning, critical reflection, reflection-in-action, reflection-on-action, self-reflection, and visual reflection), and often, no definition is provided for the concept of reflective practice. The research appears to include either students (or beginning clinicians) or expert practitioners. The most frequently used procedures for teaching reflection are reflective writing and reflective discussion, and these methods are employed in either academic or clinical settings. For the purposes of this text, we will draw, principally, from the work comprising CSD students, as opposed to practicing clinicians.

Hill et al. (2012) examine the use of reflective strategies in novice speech-language pathology students in Australia. Aiming to examine the nature of undergraduate CSD students' reflective skills, Hill et al. review reflective journal writings from 52 second year undergraduate students who participated in a clinical simulation with a standardized patient (SP). In other words, the students functioned as clinicians intent on conducting specific interviews with an actor trained to perform as the parent of a child with speech difficulties.[3] Following the interviews, the students were instructed to write a reflection on the experience in response to three questions: (1) What did I learn from this experience? (2) Given a similar situation in the future, what changes would I make to the way I managed the experience? (3) In what ways did I use my background knowledge in clinical practice to assist me in managing the situation? After coding the written reflections, the investigators found that a majority of undergraduate students use some type of reflection (94%), although very few convey critical reflection (3%), which the authors identified as being able to make changes in how one views a circumstance and/or would act at the time or if given another opportunity. Typically, reflections from beginning students are more likely to be focused on concrete elements that are direct comments on their own behaviors (Geller & Foley, 2009). Examples in which students demonstrated reflection that showed some level of critical reflection include the following statements:

> I also learnt ways of wording questions . . . in words that were easy for the parent to understand, rather than flood her with terminology that held little meaning to her. (p. 419)

> I know I should be thinking of setting their mind at ease . . . but at this stage it's difficult not to just focus on "What am I going to say." (p. 419)

The authors recommend the incorporation of reflection training into education in CSD and suggest that students at a beginning level may not yet have skill with applying already learned material to help with new learning. As well, the

---

[3]The reader should keep in mind that the academic and clinical training for clinicians in other countries may differ from what is provided in the United States.

use of reflective tasks presupposes that students have developed some level of self-direction in their learning (e.g., Sobral, 2005). These two factors (applying old material/strategies to new learning and the use of self-direction in learning) may need to be taught and fostered in the context of reflective activities. Citing research identifying barriers to the use of reflection by advanced students or practitioners (e.g., not enough time, feeling that practical experience is more valuable to learning than is academic experience; Duffy, 2009; Gallagher et al., 2017; Platzer, Blake, & Ashford, 2000), I argue that the emergence of reflective skills must be nurtured from the beginning, and for CSD students, that means taking advantage of opportunities for encouraging reflection during observation provided in the undergraduate curriculum.

As noted, CSD undergraduates are expected to complete 25 hours of supervised clinical observation, and it is during these experiences that students' skills at reflection can be cultivated. Meilijson and Katzenberger (2014) describe a CSD program in which reflective practice is introduced. Along with education and training involving case-based instruction and evidence-based practice, the program at Hadassah Academic College in Jerusalem, Israel, provides opportunity to learn about reflective practice based on Schön's (1983) concepts of "reflection-on-action" (a retrospective view) and "reflection-in-action" (a real-time view). The expectations of the students are to create a new understanding of the situation and use their new perception to inform current/future actions. Within this process, students will tie their feelings and theoretical perspectives to the task of constructing new meaning. This orientation to reflection borrows from those espoused by Boud, Keogh, and Walker (1985) in their work on the relationship between reflection and learning. According to these authors, the actions of reflection include recalling or detailing the experience, paying attention to feelings, and evaluating the experience. The complexity of these tasks is dependent on the experience and, for beginning CSD students, must be guided. Among the activities tied to clinical observation are readings on reflection, the presentation of a case example from their observation in the context of a structured, guided group meeting, and participating in simulations. Students are also required to produce written reflections on their experience. Presented below is a reflective exercise to help guide beginning CSD students while engaging in clinical observation.

A First Reflective Exercise
With a partner (preferably someone you do not know well), share a story about a time when you needed some type of health care. Listen to your partner's story. Now, on your own, briefly respond (using reflection-on-action) to the following:

1. *What was it like to tell your story?*
2. *Did you find yourself emphasizing certain aspects of your story more than others?*
3. *Did your partner ask any questions? If so, what types of questions were asked?*
4. *Did telling your story evoke familiar feelings?*

5. *Did you learn anything new or gain any new insight from having to tell your story?*
6. *What details do you remember from your partner's story? And why do you think these particular details stand out to you?*
7. *How did you find yourself responding emotionally to your partner's story?*
8. *Did you learn anything new or gain any insight from having listened to your partner's story?*

Reflective Writing and Narrative

Before one can become a reflective practitioner, one must be provided the opportunity to grow and enhance attitudinal characteristics consistent with reflective practice and to develop the necessary skills for self-awareness and self-reflection. Daaleman, Kinghorn, Newton, and Meador (2011) reason that a student, in the process of becoming a health care provider, learns self-awareness within the context of other students and mentors who share the same motivation to help the well-being of others. The formation of a professional identity is enhanced through the promotion of reflection, belonging to a community of learners, and activities, such as narrative (just like that done in the previous exercise) or reflective writing (e.g., Daaleman et al., 2011; Warmington & McColl, 2016). A considerable amount of research in health disciplines has investigated the use of reflective writing and narrative for increasing *self-awareness* (e.g., Constantinou & Kuys, 2013; Gallagher et al., 2017; Koh, Wong, & Lee, 2014), *professional identity* (Easton, 2016; Warmington & McColl, 2016), *communication* (Koh et al., 2014), and *critical thinking* skills (e.g., Naber & Wyatt, 2014). As a prelude to introducing tasks that can be used to foster reflection through writing and narrative, we will review, briefly, the findings in the aforementioned areas (focusing on studies involving students, in general, and the discipline of CSD, if available).

Self-Awareness and Communication

Koh et al. (2014) investigate the effects of a "task-based learning experience" (preparing and presenting a public lecture on a topic in public health) on a group of medical students in an elective involving public health communication. Students record responses to the experience through journal entries in which they reflect on the activity, who they interacted with, what they contributed, and how they felt about the experience, along with integrating their own behavior change with theoretical information on health communication. Of significance is the growth that students report in terms of self-awareness, strengths and limitations, and communication skills. Likewise, Constantinou and Kuys (2013) identify similar outcomes for physiotherapy students while participating in a study of "guided reflective journal" use. In particular, the guided journal work helps students gain greater insight into how their perceptions of their patients and their own skills change over the course of a practical experience.

Professional Identity

Professional identity is often shaped through the process of sharing stories (Easton, 2016; Warmington and McColl, 2016). The literature tells us that professional identity is a fluid concept, changing and being redefined through multiple experiences involving professional interactions. Goldie (2012) notes that social, relational, and contextual factors all influence the development of a professional identity in medical students. He states, "During medical school the formation of students' professional identities are influenced more by the informal and hidden curricula than by formal teaching experiences" (e645). What is meant by this is that students use their experiences from a host of interactions to practice ways of functioning professionally, which are molded by reactions of others, feedback from mentors, and repeated interactions with colleagues. Warmington and McColl (2016) highlight the relational nature of storytelling in the process of identity formation in medical students. These researchers use an ethnographic approach, analyzing the ways in which medical students tell stories about their experiences interacting with patients. Drawing from two separate interviews with two medical students, Warmington and McColl describe the language used to make links between the student and the supervising physician (e.g., "I think doctors are more on the side of the students . . ."; "But we'd never been asked to leave a ward round by a patient—and most doctors would never give patients the option; and don't introduce us as students"). The authors use these quotes as examples of how a physician's behavior in a clinical context is part of the "hidden curriculum," and students learn to read the behaviors as models of professional identity. Integrating their findings into the larger realm of professional identity work, the authors suggest that the acquisition of a professional identity in students can be facilitated through the sharing of stories, something clinical teachers can implement with their students.

Critical Thinking

Critical thinking and reasoning skills can be promoted through reflective writing and the use of narrative tasks (Cruz, Caeiro, & Pareira, 2014; Naber & Wyatt, 2014). Naber and Wyatt (2014) examine the effects of several reflective tasks, including reflective writing, journal writing, triangulation, and faculty feedback, on the promotion of critical thinking skills in undergraduate nursing students. Comparing a group of nursing students who were asked to complete the reflective tasks to a group who did not conduct structured reflection activities, the authors find few differences between them on measures of critical thinking. A significant difference is found between the groups in "truth-seeking" behavior, which is consistent with other literature correlating the experience of writing reflectively with students learning the importance of basing clinical decisions on valid information and seeking assistance from other health care providers. Inconsistent with the research on changes in critical thinking and reflective writing activities are the nonsignificant findings of their study. Naber and Wyatt suggest that the shorter timeframe of their study, perhaps, did not give the students the time to generalize their insights from the reflective tasks.

In a study of Portuguese physiotherapy students in the fourth year of their undergraduate program, Cruz et al. (2016) present the effects of a narrative reasoning course on the students' perceptions of patient-centered care. In the course, students engage in readings and other tasks focused on two elements: the "collaborative therapeutic relationship" and "illness narratives." Using a focus group approach to collect students' input, the authors identify three themes expressed by the students: (1) the development of new or improved skills (i.e., better listening and better observing) that allow them to be more effective with their patients, particularly related to increased empathy and integrating their patients into decision-making; (2) clinical reasoning shifted from clinician focused to patient focused, which many students resisted at first; and (3) their professional identity felt challenged, largely reflecting the shift to being patient centered. Overall, the authors propose the inclusion of direct narrative reasoning content and tasks encourages the advancement of a patient-centered approach to treatment by requiring students engage in narrative activities centered on collaboration and the nature of illness from a patient perspective. Try the following exercise to help you contemplate how listening to a client's or patient's story might help you in identifying important factors to include in a therapeutic process.

In a final note, Easton's (2016) analysis of narratives delivered in medical school lectures finds a much larger quantity than expected; that is, medical school lecturers use narratives in their teaching more than they perceive they do. Most students (but not all) find narratives particularly helpful in facilitating the recall of information, creating a context in which to engage with and better understand material. Easton also suggests the use of narrative for encouraging professional identity and helping students make connections to the "human" side of medicine through promoting empathy. Next time you find yourself in class (CSD or other), pay attention to how often the instructor uses narratives or stories to reinforce the material. Do you think narratives can be an effective tool for professors to use when facilitating students' learning of complex concepts or material?

A Second Reflective Exercise
Watch the first 15 minutes of the Jon video during which he responds to the clinician's inquiry about why he sought out treatment. In writing, complete the following:

1. The most important feature of this video clip is . . . .
2. I wish I knew more about . . . .
3. If I were the clinician, I would . . . .

Now, write a paragraph on how observing this video clip and responding to the prompts have helped you reflect (or not). Share your responses with your class. Write about how being able to discuss each person's impressions helps with developing reflection skills.

Group Process

A group experience interwoven with reflection appears to enhance learning, and the group process has been studied in relation to its effect on the development of reflection skills. In a study of midwifery students in Ireland, Gallagher et al. (2017) note that the most significant positive effects of the participation in group reflection are: overall support among peers, enhancement of learning, and the opportunity to link theory to practice. While the students preferred a less structured approach to the group sessions, they recognized the value of having a formalized guide to reflecting. Moreover, they expressed support for developing a culture of confidentiality and trust such that they felt free to share in the group. These components, provided by mentors or group facilitators, can be co-constructed by both students and mentors.

Another example of the use of group process in facilitating reflection comes from work done with medical students involved in clinical situations demanding strong communication skills. Lutz, Roling, Berger, Edelhäuser, and Scheffer (2016) investigated the use of a group reflection paradigm for improving the creativity of medical students' responses to complex clinical communication situations. Their system for evaluating creativity included a model drawn from the work of Rhodes (1961), which characterizes creativity along four dimensions: product, process, person, and place (the "4 P's model"). This framework, as illustrated by Lutz et al., is presented in Table 3–3. Summarizing the outcomes of their study, Lutz et al. indicate the "product" involved the emergence of new and creative solutions to communication situations students described as challenging. As an example, the authors provide the following quote from one such student:

Well, it was a difficult situation for me . . . and it was actually a real relief that . . . such a specific possible solution was developed, one that I could implement and that then also, at least for me, really brought a sense of finding inner peace in this insoluble situation. (p. 303)

In terms of "process," students commented that reflective practice had a positive impact on their own growth in reflection, helped them achieve a better capacity to appreciate others' concerns, and allowed them to see how creativity could be used to solve problems. The authors state that, with repeated experience, the students came to see reflection as a "tool" for continuing clinical practice. Development in creativity relative to "person" was observed in how students reflected on their own sense of self (e.g., "I personally see this as the difference between feeling powerless and overwhelmed and a certain competency that can be achieved over time," p. 304). And, finally, Lutz et al. (2016) report that, with "place," students used the combination of real clinical circumstances and reflection to form their autonomous professional selves. For instance, in approaching a complex situation in which clear answers are not apparent, rather than ignoring, dismissing, or downplaying the dilemma, the students learned the value in stepping back and reflecting to allow for creative problem solving. They found the use of their own clinical experiences, reflecting on them, and determining possi-

Table 3–3. Characteristics of the Combined Creativity Framework

4 P's	Characteristics
Product	A product is creative when it is "new" and "useful"
Process	Problem finding: Recognizing that a problem exists, finding gaps, inconsistencies, or flaws
Preparation	Preparatory phase: Gathering and reactivating relevant information
Incubation	Divergent thinking: Broad attention, or associative thinking: generating alternative ideas
	Ideas churn around below the threshold of consciousness
Illumination	Aha moment, insight occurs, often not one single moment
Elaboration	Convergent thinking: Evaluating. Refining and developing one's idea
Person	Willingness to overcome obstacles and perseverance, willingness to tolerate ambiguity, openness toward experiences and complexity, self-efficacy, increased motivation
Place (creativity fostering environments)	Presence of challenge and autonomy, social interaction and support

Source: Adapted from Lutz, Roling, Berger, Edelhäuser, and Scheffer (2016).

ble solutions vital to seeing themselves as capable. Ultimately, the group context provided support and expansion of perspectives that facilitated problem solving and skill acquisition. Referring to the group process, one student remarked, "The others always have an external view of the situation and can bring this in, something that always really helped me personally, introducing new aspects and possible solutions" (p. 306).

In summary, self-reflection is something that takes time and is continually developing throughout one's career (and life). As we practice reflecting, we get better at it, but there are certain experiences and activities that can enhance our learning of self-reflective skills. The research tells us that having an opportunity to explore experiences through reflective writing and receiving feedback on that writing enhances growth in reflective skills. Moreover, sharing observations and clinical experiences with peers (both from the same discipline and in an interdisciplinary forum) goes a long way toward increasing confidence and communication skills, which help to create a reflective practitioner. In addition to exploring these processes through the exercises presented within this chapter, further activities are included at the end.

Critical Thinking

Critical thinking involves asking questions and assessing the quality of the answers using reasoning and evidence, rather than anecdotes, emotions, or beliefs.

As articulated by Finn (2011) in his description of the relationship between critical thinking and evidence-based practice, there is intent on the part of the thinker ". . . to engage in an evaluative process that is based on a set of skills that results in justifiable decisions that can be applied for promoting human change" (p. 70). The development and active advancement of critical thinking skills are key to becoming an effective clinician. In fact, it has been argued that critical thinking be explicitly designated as a core competency that health care providers must achieve (Papp et al., 2014). Papp and her colleagues suggest that, "Because it underlies performance in other competency domains, critical thinking can be considered a 'metacompetency,' or a set of attributes that are necessary for one to attain mastery across multiple competency domains" (p. 717). The American Speech-Language-Hearing Association (ASHA), as well as many other professional organizations, has endorsed and promoted critical thinking as a core competency for audiologists and SLPs (ASHA, 2004, see also ASHA, 2015; Council for Clinical Certification in Audiology and Speech-Language Pathology, 2013). Certainly, it is unlikely we would come across an individual or an organization that does not believe that critical thinking skills are foundational to quality practice. That said, we need to ask what, exactly, are critical thinking skills and how do we acquire them? Are we simply born with the capacity for thinking critically and by virtue of enduring an educational or training program, we come out with a fully developed mechanism for critical thinking? Not likely! Rather, although we know that the best critical thinkers are taught specific skills and provided opportunities to practice them (e.g., Abrami et al., 2008), we also know there are certain "dispositions" that are related to critical thinking. In determining the essence of critical thinking for the purposes of reflecting on one's own abilities and facilitating its acquisition, we turn to Wade, Tavris, and Garry (2014), who outline features of critical thinking. Among these are (1) a desire to engage in critical thinking, (2) a set of necessary skills, (3) a specific goal to determine if certain information is acceptable, (4) evaluation of what is known must be verified using appropriate supportive material, rather than emotional or anecdotal information, (5) critical thinking is understood to be neutral in that engaging in it is not meant to be an attack on someone who is presenting an issue or problem, and (6) critical thinking should always move forward and be used to advance humanity. Finn et al. (2016) point out that affective components, that is, emotions, should not be disregarded when it comes to critical thinking. In fact, with audiology and SLP, emotion plays a significant role because it is how we feel about our work and our clients/patients that truly prompt us to use critical thinking and evidence-based practice processes in providing the best possible treatment for our clients/patients.

In addition to the features presented above, there is an understanding that effective critical thinkers possess characteristics that serve the process of critical thinking. Through the development of their California Critical Thinking Dispositions Inventory, Facione and colleagues (Facione, Facione, & Giancarlo, 2000; Facione, Facione, & Sanchez, 1994) identified a set of dispositions demonstrated to be central to effectual critical thinking. These are featured in Table 3–4.

Table 3–4. Dispositions to Think Critically

Disposition	Definition
Inquisitiveness	One's intellectual curiosity and desire for learning
Open mindedness	Being tolerant of divergent views and sensitive to the possibility of one's own bias
Systematicity	Being orderly, organized, focused, and diligent in inquiry
Analyticity	Prizing the application of reasoning and use of evidence to resolve problems, anticipating potential conceptual or practical difficulties, and consistently being alert to the need to intervene
Truth seeking	Being eager to seek the best knowledge in a given context, courageous about asking questions, and honest and objective about pursuing inquiry even if the findings do not support one's self interests or one's preconceived opinions
Self-confidence	Trusting the soundness of one's own reasoned judgments and leading others in the rational resolution of problems
Maturity	Approaching problems, inquiry, and decision making with a sense that some problems are necessarily ill-structured, some situations admit more than one plausible option, and many times, judgments must be made on standards, contexts, and evidence that preclude certainty

Source: Adapted from Walker (2003).

Consistent with those of Wade et al. (2014), these dispositions present a picture of a thinker who is systematic, recognizes her or his strengths (confident), desires truth and an expanded understanding of issues, and is capable of engaging in appropriate reasoning that takes into consideration that many outcomes of a critical process may be ambiguous. As an individual who is intent on developing sound critical thinking skills, a student in CSD will want to conduct a personal examination of the dispositions proposed in Table 3–4 and seek opportunities to practice applying them. The obtaining of observation hours is an excellent time for this type of practice. Several activities designed to incorporate critical thinking are included in the exercise section at the end of the chapter, but I present one here as a way of getting us thinking about critical thinking!

A Critical Thinking Exercise
Take each of the dispositions described in Table 3–4 and jot down an example in which you displayed that disposition. Consider using this listing when conducting clinical observation, can you find examples in which a clinician demonstrated the disposition? Just for fun, listed below are two examples from my own experience.

> *Inquisitiveness—when I decided to return to school for a PhD, my academic advisor asked what area of the field I intended on studying. I replied, "I just want to study it all again, just at a higher level." She informed me that wasn't*

how typical PhD degrees were pursued, and eventually, I did have to settle on a major area study—but the truth was, I really was curious and wanted to learn it all again!

Truth-seeking—I once worked with a gentleman seeking treatment for stuttering. After several weeks of therapy, it seemed we had reached an impasse; progress was elusive and my client expressed dissatisfaction. I could have responded with reminding him of his responsibilities in the therapeutic process or suggested we increase our efforts, but what I chose to do was ask him directly how he was feeling about the therapeutic process and the therapeutic relationship. He replied by sharing with me his discomfort with the therapy thus far and his desire to work with a male clinician. Had I not been willing to seek out the truth from my client, the process may have stagnated even further and our relationship deteriorated. As it turns out, I was able to refer him to a local male SLP and we both felt positive about the outcome.

Figure 3–1 illustrates the three components that represent the process of critical thinking (as diagrammed by Finn et al., 2016). Initially, the practitioner must *interpret* the information available. As an example, if one is provided a "working diagnosis" of a client/patient prior to conducting an evaluation, the audiologist or SLP will want to determine how much she or he knows about the situation, including the referral source and the diagnosis. Second, the practitioner engages in

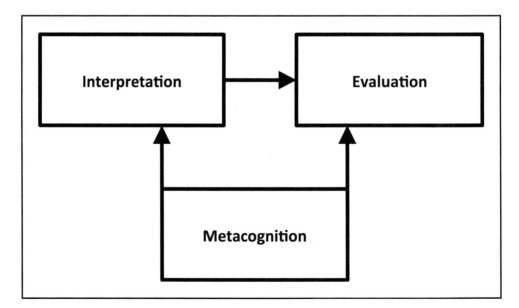

Figure 3–1. Three interactive stages that form the basis of critical thinking skills. Reprinted with permission from Finn, P., Brundage, S.B., & DiLollo, A. (2016). Preparing our future helping professionals become critical thinkers: A tutorial. *Perspectives of the ASHA Special Interest Groups (SIG 10), 1,* 43–68.

a process of *evaluating* the suitability of the information being interpreted. In other words, the SLP or audiologist will want to know upon what evidence the proposed diagnosis is based and how plausible that evidence is for the diagnosis. Eventually, the clinician must make a judgment about the credibility and applicability of the evidence for her or his own circumstances. A third component of critical thinking is that of *metacognition*. In this phase of critical thinking, the practitioner is reflecting on her or his own process of thinking—how well does she or he understand the issue? Has she or he reflected on her or his own biases, assumptions, or values relative to the issue? And, has the clinician applied different thinking strategies to the issue in order to determine the most appropriate and effective approach?

So, now that we have a basic notion of what critical thinking means, let us contemplate how these skills are gained and how best to use them in clinical practice. Table 3–5 shows the developmental milestones generated by a subcommittee of educators in health professions following a 2011 conference examining the state of critical thinking in health care disciplines (Papp et al., 2014). We will explore these "stages" as a way of helping us appreciate our own acquisition of this important way of thinking. To begin with, it is important to recognize a few suppositions connected with the work conducted by the group outlining the developmental milestones. First, they remind us that not all thinking is necessarily critical thinking. Many people rely on forms of thinking that could be considered more "automatic" or less well grounded in foundational principles. A second point they make is that the types of thinking that go into problem solving may very well be constrained or determined by the context or setting in which the problem is being confronted. This points directly to the challenge of not only identifying the critical thinker and the strategies she or he uses but also how one assesses the process of critical thinking.

Even with the difficulties in determining the exact types of thinking or contextual influences on thinking, we see from the information in Table 3–5 that novice thinkers differ from advanced and accomplished thinkers in many ways. The novice thinker has yet to develop any skill in reflecting on her or his own thinking as well as that of others. The "unreflective thinker" in CSD is likely to be early in her or his academic program and relies on word-for-word information from professors to be "the truth." At this point in the evolution toward becoming a CSD professional, the student often has difficulty with the many aspects of "gray" in the field. Why is there not one proven approach to treating language delay in preschool children? How is it that we can observe the same clinician working with the same client on multiple occasions and see entirely different interactions? How come this hearing aid fits and works well with yesterday's client, but not with today's, who has a similar audiogram? It is not uncommon for students at this developmental level to rely in large measure on the memorization of factual information or personal experience. As we move along in our advancement, the ability to think more deeply emerges. An undergraduate student in CSD is continually building a knowledge base of the field at the same time she or he is developing global thinking skills. Presumably, these skills are progressing as a result of the larger learning environment within the college or university

Table 3–5. Stages in Development of Critical Thinking

Stage	Description
1. Unreflective thinker	
Metacognition	Does not examine own actions, thinking. Unaware of thinking processes in self or others.
Attitudes	Lacks flexibility, difficulty accepting ambiguity. Uses current beliefs, does not make use of feedback.
Skills	Single approach to problem solving. Uses old strategies for gathering and understanding information.
2. Beginning critical thinker	
Metacognition	Becomes aware of different ways of thinking and begins thinking critically. Needs external motivations.
Attitudes	Does not seek feedback, but open to it. Willing to accept other clinician's conclusions without examining evidence.
Skills	At risk for bias because of influence of own experience—"availability bias."
3. Practicing critical thinker	
Metacognition	Learner is familiar with metacognitive theories, conscious effort in own critical thinking.
Attitudes	Demonstrates humility in acknowledging uncertainties, open to challenges about own thinking, welcomes new approaches.
Skills	Uses principles to make sense of observations and guide decisions.
4. Advanced critical thinker	
Metacognitive	Uses numerous approaches to critical thinking, recognizes the importance of critical thinking. Regulates and seeks to improve critical thinking skills.
Attitudes	Actively seeks out feedback, demonstrates interest in learning new approaches to thinking.
Skills	Uses both analytical and intuitive strategies to solve problems, adjusts thinking to be appropriate to the context.
5. Accomplished critical thinker	
Metacognitive	Uses theories of metacognition to improve conceptualization of problems, is in charge of own thinking, revises and uses strategies to enhance thinking.
Attitudes	Works to improve own thinking as well as others', recognizes own biases, is creative in approaching problem solving.
Skills	Switches between analytical and intuitive strategies adeptly, sees complexity of situations, can create new knowledge.

Source: Adapted from Papp et al. (2014).

experience. The reading, writing, and thinking done in other classes all serve to enhance overall skill with critical thinking. What is important for the later application of knowledge and skill in the discipline is that the student recognizes her or his thinking processes—the acquisition of a "meta" approach to thinking and problem solving. For this text, it is hoped that students engaging in clinical observation have reached a point at which they can begin to examine how it is they interpret and evaluate information gleaned through observation, what biases or assumptions they hold, how they handle feedback, and what skills or strategies they have when problem solving during the observation process. Students should continually strive toward advanced and accomplished critical thinking, and at the same time, they need to recognize that an advanced approach to thinking and problem solving not only requires much knowledge, practice, and experience, it also necessitates certain attitudes and dispositions. See the examples in Tables 3–6 and 3–7 to better understand the developmental process in critical thinking.

A process for assisting CSD students in honing their critical thinking skills has been presented by Finn (2011) and colleagues (Finn et al., 2016), which draws from work done by Browne and Keeley (2015). These authors suggest that the best place to start a process of critical thinking is to pose the right question. In developing a process of critical thinking, we will want to pose questions that assist us in interpreting and evaluating the material in front of us, as well as help us frame further understanding. Initially, a clinician will want to address the "WHAT" of a circumstance. That is, what does the information constitute? As the clinician, we want to know what issue is at hand and whether any conclusion can be drawn. Further, we want to make ourselves aware of any preconceived ideas or assumptions and the presence of any content that may be unclear. Once we are comfortable with our interpretation, we move on to evaluating the information. Evaluation is a method of determining the rigor and appropriateness of the material. As stated, "How good is the evidence?" During this process, the practitioner is identifying the reasons why the information or claim is being presented, whether or not those reasons are valid, and how solid is the evidence. An example scenario might be a case in which a classroom teacher is arguing for central auditory testing on a youngster in his class. The audiologist, in addition to interpreting the referral, must evaluate the reasons why the teacher believes that a central auditory processing disorder (CAPD) is present, the type and validity of evidence being presented by the teacher, along with other potential explanations. In this case, the audiologist is going to want to review the research to maintain her or his own informed perspective.

Finally, the metacognitive process is the time when the practitioner examines her or his own thinking. Finn et al. (2016) suggest three steps in the metacognitive process when implementing evidence-based practice. First, the clinician examines her or his own understanding of the issue. So, in the case of the teacher recommending central auditory testing, the audiologist will want to make sure that both she or he and the teacher have a shared understanding of what constitutes CAPD and the characteristics the teacher is observing in the child that led to the referral. Second, the clinician must examine her or his own biases or assumptions. So, perhaps, the audiologist is skeptical about a teacher's ability to recognize symptoms

Table 3–6. Stages in Development of Critical Thinking: A Speech-Language Pathology Example by Patrick Finn Ph.D.

Speech-language pathology scenario:
Amarantha Smit, a healthy 2-year, 6-month old girl, is referred for speech and language assessment. The mother is concerned that she may be exhibiting stuttering. The mother claims that her child's speech is occasionally characterized by multiple syllable repetitions (e.g., "if-if-if-if-if") and incomplete syllable repetitions (e.g., "ca-ca-ca-can"). The mother reports that Ama appears to be mildly frustrated about her speech during these moments. During the assessment, none of these behaviors is evident in the child's speech. Her speech and language appear to be age appropriate. In fact, her language skills may be slightly above her age level. There is no reported family history of stuttering or other communication disorders.

Unreflective thinker: "This sounds like an unambiguous case of normal developmental disfluencies. The fact that I didn't see any stuttered speech behaviors suggests that the mother is overly concerned and misdiagnosing her child's behavior. The fact that there is no family history of stuttering reinforces this conclusion. I would recommend dismissing this case."

Interpretation	Metacognition	Attitudes	Skills
The thinker jumps immediately to the most obvious diagnosis and does not consider other possibilities.	The thinker appears to be unaware of the possible fallibility in the diagnostic process and fails to acknowledge the possibility that there may be other possible explanations.	The tone of certainty suggests that she is closed to considering other possibilities.	Her thinking is reflexive in that she selects those characteristics that are consistent with a "textbook" description of normal developmental disfluencies. But she ignores the other facts that suggest that stuttering is still a likely possibility.

Beginning critical thinker: "Amarantha is a healthy normally developing child. I was unable to see any evidence of stuttering speech behavior during my assessment. Therefore, I'm leaning toward the possibility of normal developmental disfluencies. The fact that the child's language skills are above her age level suggest that speech motor abilities are unable to match her advanced language skills. Still, the mother's description of Ama's speech behaviors and her reactions to them are characteristic of stuttering. So I should not rule out the possibility that this is early childhood stuttering. Let's ask the mother to see if she could obtain a recording of Ama's speech at home before we dismiss this case entirely."

Interpretation	Metacognition	Attitudes	Skills
This thinker has considered additional information that raises the possibility of other diagnoses.	Although the learner considers other diagnoses, the strategies used to arrive at each do not lead to a conclusion about which possibilities are most likely.	This thinker demonstrates openness to other possibilities rather than jumping to a textbook diagnosis.	She demonstrates that she is willing to be open minded and consider the mother's diagnosis of stuttering by requesting a home recording.

Table 3–6. *(continued)*

Advanced critical thinker: "This is an interesting case of a young child who may be exhibiting early childhood stuttering based on the speech behaviors described by the mother. But it also possible that it may be normal developmental disfluencies. The fact that I was unable to see any evidence of the speech characteristics for myself raises some doubts in my mind, but that doesn't necessarily mean the mother is incorrect. The absence of evidence does not necessarily mean evidence of absence. Stuttered speech behaviors can be highly variable across time and speaking conditions. Further, the mother has seen much more of the child's behavior than I have, and thus, her concern should not be taken lightly. The mother's indication that Amarantha appears frustrated during these moments that she describes as stuttering should also be considered. A tentative diagnosis of early childhood stuttering seems warranted. Further, some of the other features mentioned—no family history, better than age-level language skills, a young female—suggest that this child may be a likely candidate for natural recovery from stuttering. Let's ask the child to return in 6 months, provide the parent with some concrete suggestions on how to respond to her child's disfluencies, and ask the parent to contact us if the symptoms increase in frequency or severity in the meantime. If the child is indeed still stuttering, the window of opportunity remains good for addressing the problem with some well-established, evidence-based treatment approaches."

Interpretation	Metacognition	Attitudes	Skills
This thinker's approach to this case is much broader than the other two with multiple possibilities being considered and the various types of evidence being weighed accordingly.	The individual understands the fundamentals of thinking about one's own mental processes and acknowledges her risk of being biased because of the lack of first-hand, observable evidence.	The thinker is acknowledging the need to be open to the possibility that the mother may be correct and is open to the as-yet-unseen alternatives.	This person weighs the various types of evidence presented. She considers the possibility of her cognitive bias and its impact on this scenario. She is considering all of the possibilities and considering different courses of action and the evidence that might support them.

Table 3–7. Stages in the Development of Critical Thinking: An Audiology Example by Patrick Finn Ph.D.

Audiology scenario:
Calvin Jacques, a middle-aged factory worker, is referred for an audiology assessment. He complains of unilateral hearing loss and occasional ringing in his ears. He mentions that he has been feeling more tired than usual and is experiencing more headaches than normal.

Unreflective thinker: "I conducted an audiological evaluation and confirmed that there is a high frequency sensorineural hearing loss. This kind of loss is consistent with a noise-induced loss given his work setting. I would recommend a hearing aid."

Interpretation	Metacognition	Attitudes	Skills
The thinker jumps immediately to the most obvious diagnosis and does not consider other possibilities.	The thinker appears to be unaware of the possible fallibility in the diagnostic process and fails to acknowledge the possibility that there may be other possible explanations.	The tone of certainty suggests that she is closed to considering other possibilities.	The thinking is reflexive in that she selects those characteristics that are consistent with a "textbook" description of a sensorineural loss and a factory work setting. But she ignores the other facts that suggest that a more serious problem may be evident.

Beginning critical thinker: "Calvin appears to have a unilateral high frequency hearing loss based on the audiogram. A word recognition test presented at a louder level, however, suggested poorer results than we might have expected. Perhaps he should discuss these findings with his doctor—especially if he has been feeling tired and experiencing headaches. Maybe we should recommend a tinnitus work up, too, given his complaint of ringing in his ears."

Interpretation	Metacognition	Attitudes	Skills
This thinker has considered additional information that raises the possibility of other diagnoses.	Although the learner considers other diagnoses, the strategics used to arrive at each do not lead to a conclusion about which possibilities are most likely.	This thinker demonstrates openness to other possibilities rather than jumping to a textbook diagnosis.	She demonstrates that she is willing to be open minded about a different diagnosis based on the additional testing.

Advanced critical thinker: "This is an interesting case of a middle-aged man who complains of a unilateral hearing loss. The audiogram confirms that there is evidence of a high frequency loss in one ear. This kind of loss would be consistent with his work setting. But I don't want to let that information override any other information. I can't ignore that the results of word recognition testing were not consistent with the audiogram. I think it would be prudent to run additional tests. Auditory brainstem response and otoacoustic emissions tests would seem warranted here. I'm especially concerned about Calvin's reports of fatigue and increased frequency of headaches. These could be signs of a more serious neurological issue, such as a tumor of the eighth cranial nerve or brainstem. We should also make sure there is a follow-up with an otolaryngologist."

Table 3–7. *(continued)*

Interpretation	Metacognition	Attitudes	Skills
This thinker's approach to this case is much broader than the other two, with multiple possibilities being considered, and the various types of evidence being weighed accordingly.	The individual understands the fundamentals of thinking about one's own mental processes and acknowledges her risk of being biased because of the work setting information.	The thinker is acknowledging the need to be open to the possibility that there may be additional concerns, and is open to as-yet-unseen alternatives.	This person weighs the various types of evidence presented. She considers the possibility of her biased assumptions and its impact on this scenario. She also constructs a reasonable case for additional testing that would determine the likelihood of other possible concerns.

of CAPD or the usefulness in testing for this disorder. She or he will need to examine the bases for her or his skepticism in order to engage in critical thinking about the teacher's concerns and request. The third step in metacognition, as described by Finn et al., is the use of appropriate strategies for achieving critical thinking. In our example, the audiologist may employ a process of open-mindedness or adjustments to her or his thinking to reflect the context. In describing the process of critical thinking, I have argued for the "thinker" to reflect on what types of knowledge she or he is relying upon and the strength, validity, and reliability of that knowledge. In the next section, the "ways" in which we "know" things are discussed to help us in our quest to hone and use critical thinking skills.

Ways of Knowing with Marisue Pickering, Ed.D.

Part of developing self-reflection skills involves examining how it is we know what we know. Some maintain that without understanding the nature of knowledge and how it fits with the larger clinical picture, implementing evidence-based practice will be difficult (Knight & Mattick, 2006). Knight and Mattick (2006) also argue that the notion of "knowledge" must go beyond scientific concepts and embrace client/patient and clinician understandings. The combination of both the practitioner perspective and the patient/client perspective is at the heart of the biopsychosocial approach; as articulated by Engel (1997), "With respect to the patient's verbal report of an illness experience and the doctor's version thereof, both constitute claims to knowledge about what each believes he/she knows about what happened and about what the patient's experiences were like. These constitute the data on which the doctor depends for further study and decision-making" (p. 524).

There are myriad "ways of knowing," some of which we will discuss here as they relate to communication and impairments of communication (see Figure 3–2). Words of caution: Ways of knowing overlap; they are not necessarily

(1) Received knowledge	An unimpeachable source told me.	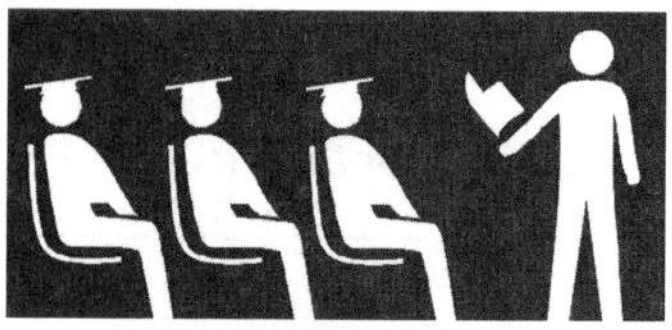
(2) Experiential knowledge	Been there, done that.	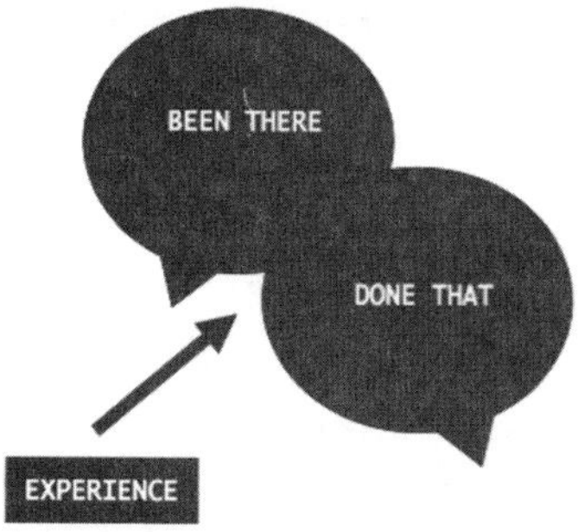
(3) Subjective knowledge	Internal process, "gut" feeling. Thought it, intuited it, interpreted it.	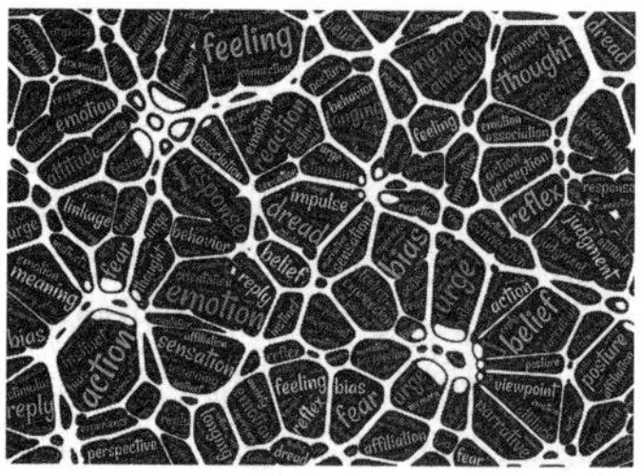
(4) *Judgmental knowledge*	Used a set of external standards.	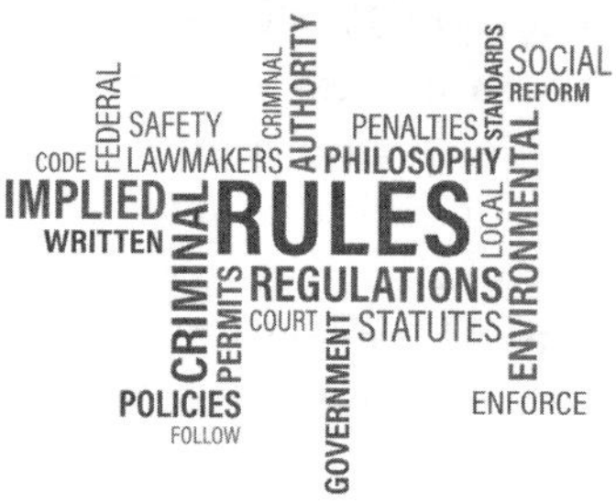
(5) *Adversarial knowledge*	Two or more people argue issues/data, "claim" to truth emerges, sometimes third party involved.	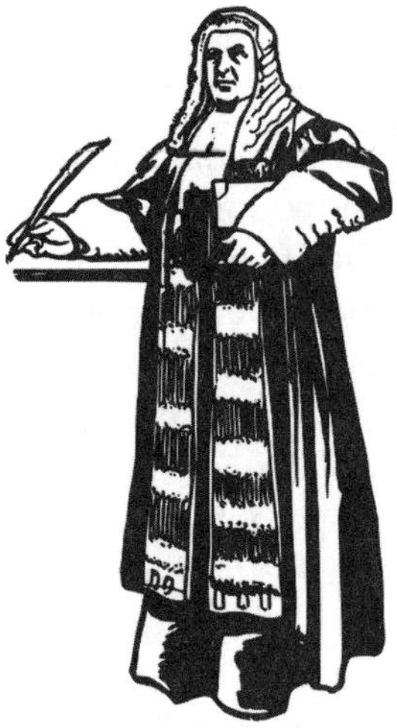

Figure 3–2. Ways of knowing.

(6) *Modus operandi*	Use habitual procedure to arrive at claim.	**M.O.**
(7) *Scientific knowledge in Natural Sciences*	Follow traditional process of scientific method.	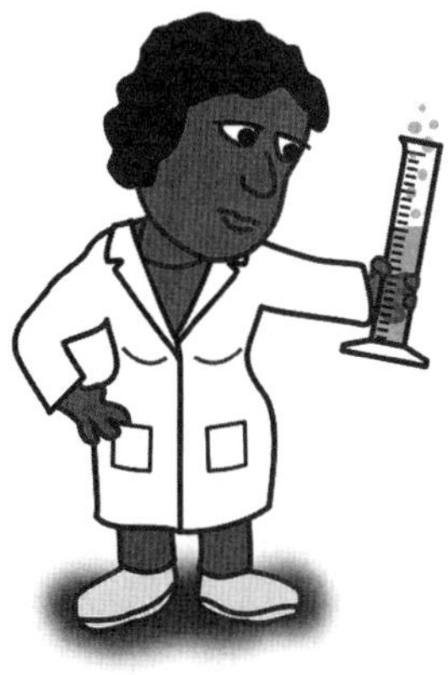
(8) *Scientific knowledge in Human Sciences*	Using definable method, seek narrative patterns.	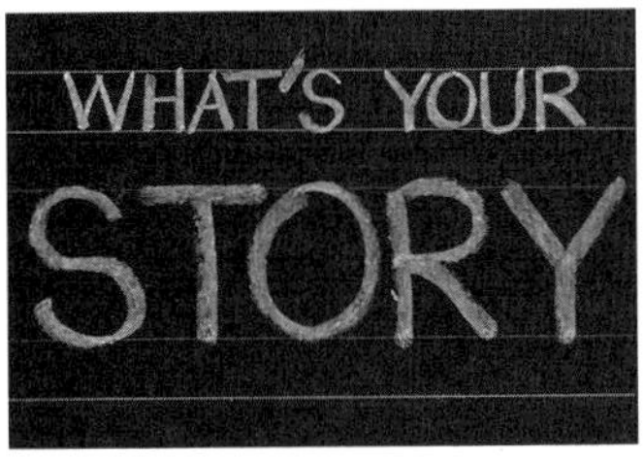
(9) *Theoretical knowledge*	Use logic, data to develop theory.	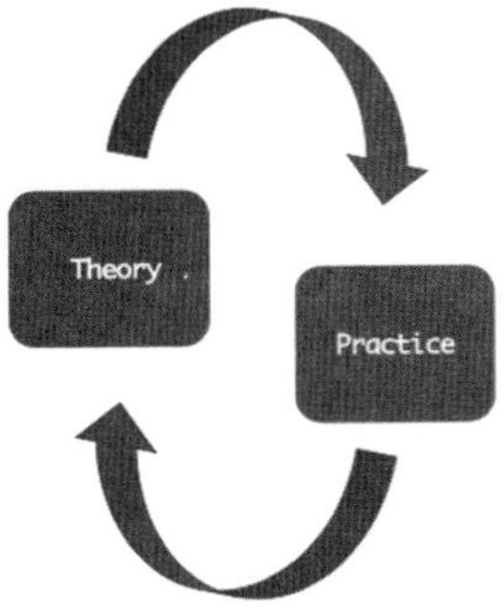
(10) *Connected/ collaborative knowledge*	Co-constructed truth or approach with others.	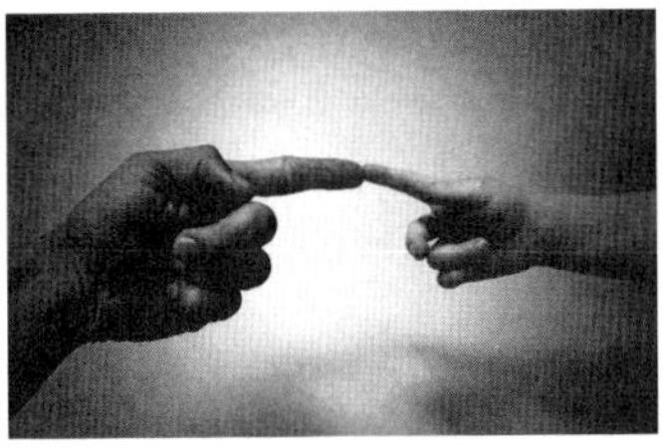

Figure 3–2. (continued)

discrete categories. In this chapter, we present them as such because it is easier to think about them in this way. Further, we all depend on a range of ways to know and understand our worlds. We base our decision making on a variety of factors, a variety of claims to knowledge. And finally, we make no assertion that this is an inclusive list of our disparate ways of knowing. As all of us experience the world, we will develop unique perspectives informed by many sources both within our culture and elsewhere. Thus, all of us possess and use our own ways of knowing. Later, in the chapter, we will explore the value of bringing together multiple ways of knowing from a variety of sources, through collaborative exercises.

Received Knowledge

Received knowledge comes from a source you trust. Someone gives you information, and you are comfortable applying it. Here one is relying on a voice of authority as the basis for decision making. Received knowledge can come from a person such as a parent, teacher, professor, doctor, religious leader, community and professional leader, politician, or even a friend. Someone tells us something, and because it is from a trusted source, we accept it as true. Received knowledge also comes from media sources we decide to trust, for example, the Web, newspapers, magazines, journals, television, talk radio, social media, and from the information presented through advertising, celebrity endorsements, journalistic reporting, and others. A trusted source can also be books such as holy books or textbooks. Or in oral cultures that tell stories more than relying on written texts, the source could be tribal stories or myths such as those that tell how the earth was created or how humans were given the gift of fire.

With received knowledge, we listen to others and accept what we are told as accurate, important, and worth remembering. As students in CSD, we learn to accept information from our textbooks, professors, professionals, and trusted online sources (e.g., ASHA website). A caution here is that the source may be incorrect or inappropriate for the current situation. A discipline such as CSD is ever evolving, with advances in research and exploration continually informing our clinical practice. Additionally, we must always recognize that different circumstances will determine different approaches in providing quality clinical services.

Experiential Knowledge

Think of this as "been there, done that" kind of knowledge. Our personal, first-hand experiences lead us to believe something is true. For example, perhaps you have been a babysitter, and this has helped you learn a lot about children; you then rely on this as acceptable knowledge in observing clinical work with children. Or your grandfather stutters, and you bring the knowledge of his experiences to observing a person who stutters.

Certain jobs place a high value on experiential knowledge; a job applicant is asked to document prior experience. A built-in assumption is that prior experience in a similar situation will help the person know how to act in a new situation. Practicum in CSD is based in part on the value of experiential knowledge. As such, the CSD student is expected to develop understanding and skill working with a variety of clients and patients in a number of different settings. Importantly, students are not left to sort it out alone. Experienced clinicians guide the student because experiential knowledge without reflection and analysis is not part of one's full clinical education experience.

As a word of caution, we must remember that we can generalize inappropriately on the basis of personal experience. We assume the new experience is exactly like the old one, and it can't be. It will be different in some way, either obvious or not. Or we assume the other person feels the way we felt in a similar situation, and they don't. We think that because something has been true in one particular situation, it is generalizable. Some elements may be, but not all.

Subjective Knowledge

We think we know something because it "feels" or seems right to us. Subjective knowledge is an individualized, internalized way of knowing. A related term might be *trusting your gut*. Subjective knowledge privileges "gut feelings" over evidence. People who have subjective knowledge are unlikely to fully explain why they hold the views they hold. Usually, the connection between subjective knowledge and the empirical, external world is not clear or straightforward. By definition, subjective knowledge cannot be proven by experiences available to everyone as it is not based on shared, verifiable facts or experiences.

Where does subjective knowledge come from? For some people, knowledge that comes from dreams, spiritual encounters, or meditative insights might fit here. Some people use the term *intuition*; others might refer to "an instinctual feeling." In part, this "intuition" comes from experience, but it also reflects our need to make sense of a world that cannot always be explained. For example, we may observe a clinical session in which a youngster is in and out of her chair multiple times. Subjectively, we might think the child is "hyper" or "noncompliant"; however, without further information, we cannot objectively understand what it is we are observing.

Although this is a way of knowing we all employ, we must recognize the pitfalls associated with it. We may ignore facts or evidence contrary to what we believe. We may overgeneralize. Because it is individualized, we don't have a way of calibrating what we know with others. Feelings are easy to manipulate, and we may not know ourselves as well as we think we do. Learning to curb our subjective interpretations is a lifelong process.

Judgment or Expert Knowledge

This is a way of knowing that comes from an expert applying a set of definable standards to phenomena. Having applied the standards, the expert makes a judgment. Although we use our five senses to obtain the evidence needed, we refer to an outer, explainable standard when the judgment is made. And it is important to note that standards change over time.

A culture will apply a set of standards in the realms of art, music, movies, dress—on and on. People who are experts judge the merits of a bottle of wine or a dog show and we have numerous articles, books, and blogs from such experts. Ways to measure or assess performance have been developed, and some are more objective than others. For example, standards applied to Olympic ice dancing appear to be more subjective than those applied to swimming.

Professions apply standards that can include the skills needed as well as the ethics expected, and judgments are made accordingly. In CSD, judgmental knowledge is used when an assessment is made about the correctness of a client's utterance. We have a definable standard by which we evaluate the outcome. Over time, a student's skill increases until a sense of competence is felt about the judgment made. A problem can arise when the standard is not understood, it is not explained before it is applied, the person applying it is inadequately trained, or it is applied differently to different people.

Adversarial Knowledge

Adversarial knowledge rests on the belief that in a disputed situation, we can arrive at an acceptable truth through balancing issues via argumentation and cross-examination. It can be viewed as a type of point–counterpoint process. This way of knowing can be seen in legal proceedings, investigative journalism, congressional hearings, and sometimes in political campaigns. In some cases, such as a courtroom, a third party (jury or judge) renders the final judgment. Usually, we expect rules or procedures to underpin the discourse.

Adversarial knowledge acknowledges that people have different perceptions, different interpretations, and different frameworks for understanding events, and as detailed analysis is applied, the best claim for truth can be determined. The assumption is that a claim for truth will emerge from the balancing of issues. In CSD, this process may take place between professionals or between clinicians and their clients, patients, or families. As an example, an SLP and a neurologist may both observe a patient with speech and language difficulties following a stroke, but they may disagree as to the nature of the difficulties. By reviewing clinical findings and debating their implications, the professionals may come to an agreement as to the primary speech and language diagnosis. The successful use of this type of process is dependent on a mutual understanding of the value of adversarial knowledge, as well as a respectful professional relationship between the parties involved.

A problem with this manner of knowing is that some people may have more data or facts than do others, and also, data can be concealed. Additionally, some people have more power or more skill, whereas some violate the rules or are adept at deception. Others may knowingly or subtly violate the rules, or the rules may be applied differently to different people. To effectively utilize adversarial knowledge, participants must share an understanding of the process.

Modus Operandi

Modus operandi (literally, way of operating) is based on the assumption that we can arrive at a claim to truth by tracking a characteristic chain of events or conditions. Following an established, unvarying, formulaic, or habitual way of operating is a way of knowing about something. For example, one might use a habitual procedure to troubleshoot a problem with a computer or a car; such a procedure might be in the form of a checklist.

Professionals use habitual procedures in the form of a specified set of tests to screen for a medical condition or a language issue, ruling out some factors, identifying others. The modus operandi used is probably based on experience or on research, and it is beneficial to know the reliability and validity of the checklist or procedure used. A technician may use modus operandi in doing her or his job; however, that individual is not expected to interpret the results of the work. SLPs and audiologists may follow procedures using this way of knowing—certainly, some clinical processes can become habitual—however, the skilled professional will recognize when modification is necessary in order to provide the best possible services. When conducting clinical observation, it is imperative that we recognize when clinical work has become routinized and active problem solving has ceased.

As indicated, this type of knowledge is mechanical. Deeper, interconnected issues and conditions as well as meanings can be overlooked. A modus operandi approach to working with people will always fall short. A physician can administer a checklist, but if she doesn't go beyond that to ask more personal questions, much can be missed. An audiologist can be quite skilled technically, but if she or he does not think to explore underlying elements and their impact, her or his client may gain only so much benefit from treatment. For example, without learning about a person's daily routine and the likely communication situations she or he may encounter, the dispensing of a hearing aid without counseling regarding its use socially may lead to less than ideal outcomes for that client/patient.

Theoretical Knowledge

Definitions of theoretical knowledge often contrast this type of knowing with hands-on, practical knowledge. Think of theoretical knowledge as a logical, carefully constructed set of explanations that you apply when trying to figure out how to act. Your theories (principles, ideas) may attempt to explain the nature of something, but theories are subject to testing, and actual verification will not have yet happened. And once some testing of the theory occurs, modification or actual denial can occur as new evidence emerges. Thus, theoretical knowledge changes and theories are created step by step. One step, one piece of evidence or logic leads to another. Theories are not sets of beliefs; they are logical explanations that have been created over time through careful observation, reasoning, or data collection.

CSD offers a good example of the use of theoretical knowledge in relation to understanding stuttering. Over the life of the field, we have had many theories about the causation of fluency problems. Also over the life of the field, researchers have collected data and validated some theories and invalidated others, based on new data collected. It is the newly informed theoretical perspective that should guide clinical work. For instance, if I espouse a theory arguing that stuttering is the result of specific parenting practices (e.g., the use of time out as discipline, or never having a consistent bed time routine), then my therapeutic approach would dictate that I work with the parents on discipline and structure. Likewise, were I to develop a theory that Brussels sprout consumption before the age of three causes hearing loss, I would counsel parents to avoid feeding their children such vegetables in early childhood.

A problem with this type of knowing is that we often hold a theory as absolute proof before it has been verified. And, of course, even in creating a theory, we may have used faulty reasoning or insufficient evidence. It is best to remind oneself that a theory can be something widely accepted because it has been borne out by fact or evidence, or it could be something closer to conjecture or hypothesis, still to be supported with sufficient data to be accepted.

Scientific Knowledge in the Natural Sciences

Scientific claims in the natural sciences rest on the principles of the scientific method that include identifying phenomena, collecting data, testing hypotheses, and analyzing results. It rests on the belief that knowledge, especially in the physical world, is confirmable (or not), through identification and manipulation of variables. Researchers carefully and methodically collect, describe, and predict physical phenomena. Analyses are often done via the application of statistical methods. Overall, a coherent and systematic structure is in place; work is not done in a chaotic or random manner. Research designs are so exact that observations can be repeated under the same conditions.

Many fields depend on this type of knowing, for example, physics, biology, and physiology. Although other ways of knowing are also used, scientific knowledge is highly valued in, for example, psychology, sociology, and CSD. Every student in CSD spends much of her or his education learning the science of the discipline. As a result, students and professionals alike rely on this type of knowing in much of their work. The processes of hypothesis testing, data collection, and interpretation are daily occurrences with each and every client or patient. One must have sophisticated scientific knowledge and facility with the scientific method in order to be successful as a CSD professional.

A caution with scientific inquiry is that it cannot be used to explain all of human behavior. Each human being is unique, and each client–clinician interaction results in unique outcomes. Thus, with traditional, natural world scientific knowledge, we run the risk of overgeneralization and bias. And we must remind ourselves that questions relating to causal factors or those pertaining to correlations will not easily be answered. Moreover, this way of knowing does not necessarily lead to personal wisdom or interpersonal empathy. We are reminded of Goldberg's "compassionate scientist," only a portion of which is determined by this type of scientific knowledge.

Scientific Knowledge in the Human Sciences

Once the scientific method became widely accepted, investigators began studying humans and the human experience. But, as alluded to, the human world can be resistive to the type of inquiry found in the natural sciences. Researchers began to understand that human experiences had fundamental differences with the natural sciences, and a field of scientific inquiry known as human sciences developed. The method often involves trained observers immersing themselves within phenomena and pulling out of this immersion important and useful data, interpretations, and conclusions.

Phenomena that might be studied include documents such as diaries, journals, or letters. The phenomena could be transcribed interviews with people, or they could be field notes of observed behavior. Data from such inquiries might resemble narratives that can be examined for patterns or video to be used for exploring interactive patterns. In CSD, we might use this type of inquiry—this way of knowing—to understand the impact of having to rely on the use of an augmentative communication system (AAC) on individuals and their loved ones, or what having a spouse with dementia means. Such explorations aim to create understanding of the phenomena. Additional human sciences inquiries might include investigating the experience of the communicative partners of people with hearing loss. In doing so, we can merge our understanding of the technical needs of a hearing aid user with the interpersonal needs of that individual's family members.

This way of knowing has the potential to produce data that could be interpreted too broadly. That is, what may be seen as an essential factor in the success of communication between an AAC user and her or his partner may not apply to all communicative partnerships involving AAC. Further, as human beings ourselves, we will always be at risk for interpreting information we collect through our own personal experiences and preferences. As suggested, it behooves us to hone our skills in the ways of knowing of both the scientific method and the human sciences.

Co-constructed or Relational Knowledge

Think of this claim to knowledge as that way of knowing that comes as a result of being in respectful dialogue with others. It means integrating knowledge from various sources, from the strengths of differing positions. It is based on an assumption that the complete truth of a person or an event is probably not going to be known; one never knows the whole story. This way of knowing means listening to others and their positions, trying to look at reality the way another person looks at it. For example, a clinician incorporates into her or his understanding how the parent experiences her or his child. The use of co-constructed knowledge is the bedrock of IPP and is essential for the delivery of the highest quality services. (See Chapter 5.)

Mediation within a conflict situation is an example of striving toward co-constructed knowledge; it is often used in divorce cases, property disputes, human rights grievances, and union negotiation. Connecting or sharing knowledge helps people enhance their understanding and allows for a reasonable and agreed-upon resolution of a situation.

A problem is that many realities interact and can conflict or contradict one another, and it can be hard to make sense of them. Also, this way of knowing takes time, sometimes a long time. Further, some people do not want to give up an adversarial or power role in order to include the views of others. This can especially be true for professionals who have invested years of education and practice into developing themselves as experts in their fields. Clinicians in CSD are reminded that their work involves other human beings, all of whom bring to the clinical relationship a different set of experiences, beliefs, and realities. If we think of our work as facilitating change, and we are change agents, then we must appreciate the perspectives of our clients, patients, and their families—these perspectives, these realities, are where we begin our work. And we cannot get started without first coming together and co-constructing our understanding of that which is to be changed and where we might be headed. The process of change begins with the development of relational knowledge. We will explore this further when we delve into the client–clinician relationship later in this book.

Culturally Sensitive Practice

Clinical practice that is culturally sensitive is the foundation for applying different "ways of knowing." One way to think about culturally sensitive practice comes from the exploration of "shared territories." Some years ago, one of us explored the construct of "shared territories," meaning that all of humanity is in the diversity mix (Pickering, 2003). This construct, borrowed from Flecha (1999), means putting aside the concept of a majority and minority, as well as discarding the notion that one person or group is the norm and everyone else is an "other." The following quote from Pickering's article reflects the overall concept:

. . . human diversity reflects the social profile of the planet—at a minimum, diversity is visible culturally, linguistically, racially. Diversity is the norm, and as embodiments of the planet's social diversity, we literally share territories of space, time, and communication. (p. 288)

Within the construct of shared territories, explored is the concept of multi-dimensionality, meaning that multiple frames of reference potentially can be applied when interpreting a particular set of phenomena. Another concept explored is that of partnership and dialogue, wherein one assumes the posture of engaging with others in order to learn and decide on solutions. And a final concept examined is that of ethnocentrism, which is a major impediment to culturally sensitive practice. Ethnocentrism assumes a mindset that one's particular culture is superior to all others. If we think of the various ways of knowing, we can see that engaging in true culturally sensitive practice includes the integration of our own perspectives with those of others. That is, we make sure that our "territories" overlap and are shared with those of the people with whom we work.

Striving to provide culturally sensitive services means we work to create an attitude of respect and a culturally safe environment. Cultural safety includes partnership, participation, and protection and upholds the cultural identity and well-being of those we serve (Oelke, Thurson, & Arthur, 2013). This means that *all* individuals have access to our services and we involve them entirely in decision making. As a result, it is believed they will engage more fully with us, which can lead to greater feelings of self-worth (Kay-Raining Bird & Eriks-Brophy, 2011).

An example of culturally sensitive/insensitive practices comes from a recent study of the Māori culture in New Zealand. In an exploration of aphasia in the Māori culture, McClellan, McCann, Worrall, and Harwood (2014) use a specific research methodology designed to best capture the experience of these indigenous people. The aim of the project was to gain insight into ". . . what makes a service culturally safe as well as 'accessible to and culturally appropriate for' Māori with aphasia and their whānau" (p. 530). Whānau refers to the individual's extended family. The approach used to collect the data is named "kaupapa Māori." This is a methodology derived within the Māori culture, which includes the analysis of power differentials and social inequalities. In the process of the study, the authors employed an advisory group (termed rangahau whānau) that was made up of Māori who had some type of experience with stroke to assist in design, participant recruitment, and advising the researchers on behavior and data analysis. Through semistructured interviews, individuals with aphasia or their whānau were asked questions about their experience with aphasia and its impact on communication. Spontaneously, many of the interviewees spoke about speech therapy, which ended up being a focus of the study. Analysis of the data identified six themes expressed by the respondents. These are illustrated in Table 3–8.

In reviewing the findings, it is important to keep in mind that the entire process of the study included the Māori rangahau whānau, who reviewed the thematic analysis and approved the quotations to be included in the article. For

Table 3–8. Six Themes Expressed About Speech-Language Therapy by Māori and Whānau

Theme	Description	Quote
"We're happy to do the work, but we can't do it alone."	Many whānau saw it as their responsibility to provide language therapy but hoped for assistance, especially knowledge and suggestions for activities/exercises.	"There is so much value for Māori people in learning how to cope after strokes, if we understand speech-language therapy techniques, and understand what they're for . . ."
Relationship	The SLP's relationship with the person with aphasia has a profound effect on the success of and satisfaction in therapy. Both positive and negative comments were received.	PWA: "She good, a lady was good to me." Interviewer: "Is that the speech therapist?" PWA: "Yeah" (head nod) "yeah."
		"You'd say, 'Oh look we're off to the hospital now, we're gonna see the speech therapist' and she was like 'oh, no, let's go to town' . . . but we'd take her up there and she was very much disinterested."
Our worldview	Recognition of culture and worldview is essential to positive, successful working alliance.	"The speech therapist didn't even consider that Mum would probably be better with cue cards that were in Māori. You know, she keeps showing 'dog,' turn the card over it say 'dog' on the back, picture of a dog. Shows it to Mum, Mum goes 'kurī' [dog] and then [SLP] goes 'no, dog.'"
Speech-language therapy setting	The therapy setting has the potential to enhance or detract and is instrumental in the relationship and the type of therapy provided. Also to be considered are community opportunities.	"You could've got around it a lot easier as a speech therapist if it was conversational and there was a fairly relaxed environment—lounge or café or anything but an office."
Aphasia resources	Most families appreciate additional resources, including exercises or opportunities for work outside of therapy. The use of appropriate resources adds to therapeutic relationships.	"The story was, I think it was about New York and ducks at New York, and my Mum, she at the time blurted out with 'But I'm from Hauiti and we have shags!' . . . You know, the context of the story that she had to read and understand, it wasn't something that she was remotely interested in at all."

Table 3–8. *(continued)*

Theme	Description	Quote
Is this is as good as it gets?	This theme is about the questions that continue for the PWA and their whānau, whether or not to continue with therapy, whether or not the person and family received enough therapy or the right therapy.	"My daughter spoke to a speech-language therapist at one stage and asked if there could be a regular monitoring of [Margaret's] progress and . . . I think she was told that no, that wasn't their modus operandi."
		"We've come to the understanding that Mum's condition is not going to get better . . . and this is as good as it gets. So we live with 'this is as good as it gets' . . . Communication-wise, we could probably try repetitively doing the cue cards and flash cards and all those sorts of things . . . we pull them out every now and again and have a go with them . . . we probably need to get better cards or more cards."

Source: Adapted from McClellan, McCann, Worrall, and Harwood (2014).

our purposes, it is vital that we recognize how the themes and quotes shed light on the therapeutic partnership. The authors' diagram illustrating how the themes interact with each other and with the relationship is pictured in Figure 3–3. The arrows shown in the diagram reflect the dynamic nature of the themes. The experience of finding ways to assist the person with aphasia and her or his family, the nature of the setting, the resources, and how we view outcome are likely to change as the relationship changes. Our role in this dynamic process is to be the facilitator while cultivating and maintaining a therapeutic relationship. If these themes are not heeded, if the clinician is not actively working on being culturally sensitive and creating a culturally safe space, the therapeutic process will be compromised. We will discuss the therapeutic relationship in greater detail toward the end of this chapter.

When it comes to providing culturally sensitive services, we need to be willing to explore our own cultures, our own backgrounds, and the environments in which we have developed. Further, the process of learning about how our own backgrounds inform our practice and interact with those of our clients/patients is an evolution from student learner to that of an experienced clinician. We will revisit the elements of culturally sensitive practice in our discussion of clinician characteristics later in this chapter and through the exercises presented at the end of the chapter.

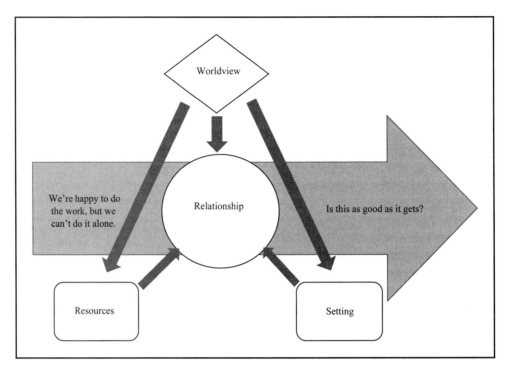

Figure 3–3. Māori and whānau experiences of aphasia. Adapted with permission from McClellan, K. M., McCann, C. M., Worrall, L. E., & Harwood, M. L. N. (2014). Māori experiences of aphasia therapy: "But I'm from Hauiti and we've got shags." *International Journal of Speech-Language Pathology, 16,* 529–540.

Professional Identity Formation

With the evolution of self-reflection skills and cultural competence, a professional identity emerges. According to Slay and Smith (2011), "Professional identity is defined as one's professional self-concept based on attributes, beliefs, values, motives, and experiences . . ." (p. 85). Foundational research in how one develops a professional self recognizes three principal influences: socialization (as in exposure to professionals and peers), adjustment during career transition, and overall life and career experiences that inform choices (Fine, 1996; Hall, 1987; Ibarra, 1999; Nicholson, 1984; Schein, 1978). For the purposes of this text, the influences of socialization and life experiences will be considered more so than career factors. The sense of self as a professional or the formulation of a professional identity is a journey, and it takes place on a continuum. Thus, for many of you, that journey is just starting. You are beginning the lifelong pursuit of continued self-awareness and reflection that will ultimately inform your clinical practice and professional identity.

In recent years, many allied health and other disciplines have spent time and energy generating lists of and implementing training in competencies believed to be the critical knowledge and skills necessary for obtaining appropriate professional credentials. Our field is one such discipline. The expected competencies for national certification in audiology and speech-language pathology are clearly articulated by the Council for Clinical Certification,[4] and in fact, our certification (the "Certificate of Clinical Competence") includes the word *competence* in its title. Of course, there needs to be a set of agreed-upon competencies that all practitioners achieving a national credential must demonstrate. That being said, it has been suggested in some professional disciplines (e.g., medicine and engineering) that the focus on fostering growth in competencies may detract from the equally important work needed for the establishment of professional identity (Jarvis-Selinger, Pratt, & Regehr, 2012; Mann, Howard, Nowens, & Martin, 2008). As per Jarvis-Selinger et al. (2012) in their argument for including professional identity work in medical education, the task of educating students should include not just "*doing* the work of a physician" but also that of "*being* a physician" (p. 1185; italics in original).

Certainly, professional identity is strongly influenced by the context and culture in which one's education takes place and the settings in which one ultimately practices. The concept of cultivating professional identity in CSD has not been well explored; however, much can be learned from examining practices in related allied health disciplines. A review of the literature in occupational therapy, physical therapy, medicine, and nursing finds a considerable number of explorations. Not surprisingly, "real-world" experience plays a part in assisting students in the process of seeing themselves as professionals (Ashby, Adler, & Herbert, 2016; Kururi et al., 2016; Lindquist, Enghardt, Garnham, Poland, & Richardson, 2006; Marañón & Pera, 2015). This is just as true for beginning students as it is for those transitioning into clinical practice. And as previously mentioned, "socialization" presents as a recurring theme among all allied health disciplines in relation to the emergence and cultivation of professional identity. Experience with socialization may take the form of job shadowing (Carey & Miller, 2011), engaging in teamwork or collaborative activities (Kururi et al., 2016), or through direct mentoring by supervisory personnel (Lindquist et al., 2006; Marañón & Pera, 2015).

On top of real-world practical experience and social interaction, communication has come to be recognized as essential to professional identity. Through the acquisition of competent communication skills, students gain confidence. Black et al. (2010) maintain that communication, because of its fundamental impact on self-confidence, may be a cornerstone to enabling professional identity. They define confidence as "a state of increasing awareness of abilities and competence (including trust in clinical decisions) as perceived by oneself and others" (Black et al., 2012, p. 1765). In their study of physical therapy students, both the

---

[4] http://www.asha.org/Certification/AboutCertificationGenInfo.htm

students and their supervisors found that expanded involvement and practice in communicating led to greater capacity to connect with patients and coworkers. So compelling is the conviction that communication is pivotal to developing healthy, beneficial, and valuable patient–/client–clinician relationships that most medical and allied health associations, worldwide, have included directives that academic programs explicitly teach such skills to their students and future professionals. In her keynote address to the 2013 American Academy of Communication in Healthcare conference in Montreal, Canada (reprinted in the journal *Patient Education and Counseling*, 2015), Deveugele highlights the centrality of communication to all health care endeavors by reminding us that instruction in and enrichment of "*personal reflection* on own communicative actions and *interdisciplinary collaboration*" [italics in original] are the responsibility of academic and training institutions (p. 1290). At the same time, she identifies the critical need for providing a "toolkit" of skills for students and professionals.

Recent explorations of communication skill development in medical students and novice physicians show an interesting interaction between direct training, social expectations, and perspective on oneself as a professional (Bombeke et al., 2011, 2012). In a series of studies examining the effects of communication training on medical students' clinical skills and attitudes, namely, "patient centeredness," researchers at the University of Antwerp in Belgium discovered that students who received direct training actually showed decreases in patient-centered attitudes, as measured by a variety of scales and questionnaires, in comparison to students who did not receive training (Bombeke et al., 2011). They interpret the findings as indicative of a gap between the "idealistic" nature of the training and the difficulty in carrying out patient-centered communication in practice. When these same researchers carried out a similar study involving early career physicians, they found a return to patient centeredness (Bombeke et al., 2012). Interviews and focus groups with the study participants led the authors to conclude that, once out from under the pressure of being evaluated (as when one is still a student), doctors are able to recall the skills learned during training and draw on them, as in a process of developing one's own clinical style. Students, on the other hand, report feeling the disconnect between what they are told to do and how their role models in the "real world" act. The authors term the evolution in patient-centered attitudes and communication a "recycle" model in that such skills appear to disappear while a student but reappear and are "recycled" when one is free to present her or his own professional style.

For CSD students, communication skills would seem self-evident. The *Standards for Accreditation for Graduate Education Programs in Audiology and Speech-Language Pathology* (Council for Academic Accreditation, ASHA, 2016a), to which educational programs are to adhere, specify that opportunities for the demonstration of "effective communication skills" must be provided to every student. Just as with other clinical professions, audiology and speech-language pathology students are expected to develop good interpersonal and communication skills, although how these are to be taught, enhanced, and evaluated is not so clear. Research on the ways in which CSD students acquire "effective communication skills" is limited, and somewhat outdated. For example, Volz, Klevans, Norton, and Putens (1978) initially found that, during clinical sessions, undergraduate speech-language pathology students show a reduced number of verbal and nonverbal behaviors that would be considered helpful or facilitative to the client–clinician relationship, even after receiving training in interpersonal communication. A follow-up study determined that SLP students could make use of training in interpersonal communication to facilitate the client–clinician relationship in the early stages of therapy. However, when compared to students from other health care disciplines who underwent more extensive training, they still demonstrated fewer facilitative responses (Klevans, Volz, & Friedman, 1981). Further, rather than using strategies that aided continuation of the conversation (such as reflecting the content or emotion expressed by the client), the SLP students relied more on what the authors characterized as "leading" responses, such as asking questions or making influencing statements. In their summary, Klevans et al. (1981) suggest that SLP students need lengthier training in communication skills.

The results of a more recent study investigating the use of SPs for training interpersonal communication skills in SLP students echo, somewhat, those of Klevans et al. (Zraick, Allen, & Johnson, 2003). Using an operationalized procedure for assessing clinical skills, which included six "interpersonal" items from the Objective Structured Clinical Examination (OSCE; Hardin & Gleeson, 1979), Zraick et al. (2003) determined that, initially, graduate student SLP clinicians performed inadequately on the interpersonal and communication items despite the fact that they showed relative competence on the other items of the OSCE. The students were provided additional education on interpersonal communication skills, after which they were rated as competent by both the SP and the faculty judges. Overall, these few reports clearly point to the importance of providing direct education and practical opportunities for learning communication skills in CSD students.

Through all of the work looking at communication skills, reflection and professional identity in medical students, allied health students and practitioners, and doctors, a few important themes emerge. As summarized by Bombeke et al. (2012), the notion of "doctor-as-person" came to the fore as paramount to learning and practicing patient-centered attitudes and communication. Accordingly, in the clinical realm, practitioners' ". . . emotions, personal histories and backgrounds, self-care and self-awareness all seem to play crucial roles" (Bombeke, 2012, p. 670). This concept is integrally related to the understanding of reflection and professional identity put forth in this text: to grow as a clinician requires both cognitive and affective processes.

Communication with clients and patients is all about establishing relationships. This is true for our professional relationships, as well. An additional area that funnels into the development of self-awareness, reflection, and professional identity is interprofessional education/interprofessional practice (IPE/IPP). Numerous sources in medicine, nursing, and other allied health disciplines tout the advantages of IPE/IPP in promoting reflection, communication, and high-quality clinical care. In her review of 50 years of literature on the interprofessional experience in medicine, Thistlethwaite (2016) reminds the reader that, although limited empirical evidence exists for the value of IPE/IPP in promoting practitioners with lasting humanistic perspectives (i.e., rigorous longitudinal studies are still to be conducted), there is strong rationale for including it early in professional education for the purposes of solidifying professional identity. Thus, in considering how CSD students begin to internalize a sense of professional identity, early exposure to IPE and experiences, coupled with opportunities to reflect, is considered vital. We will explore the integration of observation, IPE, professional identity, and reflection in the exercises presented at the end of the chapter.

Chapter Summary

This chapter has explored the first "element" of observation—you, "the observer." In it, we discuss the process of self-reflection as a means of growing as a clinician. The development of a "reflective stance"—the ability to step back, take in what has transpired, and examine our role in the process of change—is essential to acquiring and mastering clinical skills. As a result of that exploration, we know that all clinicians go through a developmental process on the way to being an expert. Also, the literature tells us that being involved with a group helps us hone the important skills, such as gaining support from professional colleagues and having the opportunity to practice critical thinking, problem solving, and linking theory to practice. We also covered the myriad ways in which we "know"—how we gain information, trust the process of learning, and develop support for our decisions. Growth as a clinician means examining our funds of knowledge and evaluating how we "know what it is we know." Finally, cultural sensitivity and communication have been considered in relation to creating an alliance with our clients, patients, families, and colleagues. These essential components are addressed further in later chapters.

Chapter Observations and Exercises

Exercise 3–1: Reflective Journal

The goal of this exercise is to develop skill at recording information from our observations and reflecting on those experiences. We will use a modified version of the SOAP note process for this journal. SOAP is an acronym that stands for subjective, objective, assessment, and plan. Most clinical health disciplines use this type of format when reporting on clients and patients. In our situation, the focus is on the observer—you! So, find yourself a mechanism that best fits your writing style in which you can record your observation SOAP notes. It can be a notebook in which you write, a tablet or laptop, even audio-dictation, as long as the end result is a written product. You will keep this SOAP reflection journal throughout the time you are observing—meaning over the course of several observations. In part, that will not only allow you to keep a log of your observations but also provide you evidence of your growth as a reflective observer. Your written journal should be organized and well written, using the following guide:

S = Subjective. This section includes your subjective thoughts and feelings.

O = Objective. This section includes any specific data you collect, the facts about the session you observed. You are not to include a full description of everything that happened. Rather, you should record the setting, persons involved, materials, and basics regarding the goals and activities attempted.

A = Assessment. This section typically includes an assessment of the success of the session. In the case of your observation and reflection, use this section to record what it is *you* gained from the observation. Consider—How successful was the experience regarding your own observation, knowledge, and skill development? Remember, this is not your assessment of the session. It is your *reflection* on the experience as an observation activity for *you*.

P = Plan. This section is your opportunity to take what you learned from this observation (i.e., your reflection on the experience) and create an informed plan for your next observation.

It is recommended that you complete this process on a series of observations over the course of a predetermined time period (perhaps a semester). At the end of the time period, identify how many hours of observation were completed and the types of conclusions you can draw given your growth and progress achieved over the course of the SOAP journal.

Exercise 3–2: Reflective Activities

A. Spend several minutes observing EB14 in our Video Library. Jot down notes—on anything. After 10 to 15 minutes, you should have a nice set of written observations. To help you reflect on the observation and what you have recorded, apply the following structure to your notes.

1. *What?*—Describe what happened, with whom, other observable elements.
2. *So what?*—Why is it important? Or is it? What is the meaning of your responses to the above question? Inferences?
3. *Now what?*—Place your observations and inferences in context. Where do they fit in the larger picture? What are the next steps? Is there more you need to learn?

B. Spend another 15 minutes observing EB14. In the course of this observation, identify two to three questions you have regarding what you have observed. Compare your questions with those of a classmate. Identify strategies for finding answers to your questions. Assign yourselves a set of the strategies to follow up on and bring together at the next class. When you come together again, review your processes for seeking the answers. Do the answers you have found inspire more questions?

C. Listen to Jon's story in our first sample from the Video Library. As an individual, note the important components you observe from this client. Get together with two or three other classmates and compare your notes. Once you have a sense of the variety, scope, complexity, and thoroughness of the group's observations, assign each of the group members one of the following roles: scribe (one to take notes on the activity), client, clinician, and observer. If you have only three members in your group, the scribe and observer will be one and the same. You will now role-play the scenario observed—in other words, you will play out what it is you just observed. So, the person who is "the client" will use Jon's information and respond with it to what the clinician might ask. The clinician, on the other hand, will want to structure the interaction with a broad perspective, as in the video. The purpose of the exercise is to give you an opportunity to experience what it might be like to share your story *as a client*. Trade roles and conduct the exercise again—keeping in mind that you don't have to make up the content, rather, with inserting yourself into the role you can embellish it with your own ideas.

In reaction to this exercise, respond to the following questions/statements:

a. What types of feelings, if any, did observing Jon's story evoke?
b. In what role did you feel more comfortable? Why do you think that is?
c. What did you notice about the players or yourself when being the observer that you didn't notice when acting in the role play?
d. How might you use this role-play experience to inform your future work as a professional?

Exercise 3–3: Ways of Knowing

For each of the items below, identify with which "way of knowing" it is associated. Once you have identified the "way of knowing," provide another example for each.

- The Earth revolves around the Sun.
- Starve a cold, feed a fever.
- After much discussion, the child's mother and the clinician decided that the reinforcement schedule being used was effective in shaping the child's behavior.
- As usual, she decided to park at the MCA because she knew there'd be an available space.
- As with the previous burglary, the criminal used the same tools to pry the office door open.
- The cook chose to include pine nuts in the casserole because they were so tasty in the rice side dish.
- The diagnostic session included evaluation of motor behaviors as well as cognition.

Exercise 3–4: Cultural Sensitivity

For an exploration of culture and health care, read the book *The Spirit Catches You and You Fall Down: A Hmong Child, Her American Doctors, and the Collision of Two Cultures* by Anne Fadiman (1997; New York: Farrar, Straus, & Giroux). Use the following comments and questions to help you reflect on the text and to promote group or class discussion.

1. Throughout the book, Hmong traditions play a central role. For example, *hu plig*, described as "soul calling," is discussed at length early in the book. Why do you suppose the author chose to relate the details and importance of this tradition? Does your family follow any traditions around the birth of a child?
2. What is the message of "fish soup" (on p. 12)? How does this relate to being a clinical service provider? How does this relate to being a client receiving services?
3. What is the significance of the history of the Hmong people? Why does the author discuss this?
4. Are there concepts, issues, ideas brought forth in this book that are unfamiliar to you? How will you learn about them?
5. How do you see this book impacting you?

Exercise 3–5: Critical Thinking

Applying Critical Thinking Skills to a Controversial Treatment Approach in Communication Sciences and Disorders by Patrick Finn

[The following is an example of an exercise in applying critical thinking skills that is based on a brief example originally described by Finn et al. (2016).]

Facilitated communication (FC) is a method claimed to help nonverbal clients with autism or other developmental disabilities to communicate. It has also been referred to as "supported typing" (Lilienfeld, Marshall, Todd, & Shane, 2014), and a variant of this approach called "rapid prompting method" has appeared more recently (Tostanoski, Lang, Raulston, Carnett, & Davis, 2014). Facilitated communication is based on the hypothesis that this approach can assist individuals in overcoming their neuromotor difficulties for making their selection of typed letters or other targets for communication by receiving physical support by a trained facilitator. An important premise of this method is that the facilitators do not assist the communicators in making their actual selections for communication. They only stabilize the communicator's hand, wrist, or arm during typing and pull it back after the selection is made (Biklen, 1992; Crossley, 1992). Not long after it appeared, FC received positive media attention when it was claimed that this method allowed many clients to reveal remarkable cognitive and communication abilities that had not been previously identified or uncovered (e.g., Crossley, 1992). But, it subsequently fell out of favor during the 1990s when research strongly suggested that the facilitated messages were being produced unwittingly by the facilitators and not the clients (Mostert, 2001). As a result, several professional associations, including ASHA (1995), wrote policy statements discouraging the use of this method. In recent years, however, there has been a resurgence in the use of FC especially with persons across the autism spectrum (Lilienfeld et al., 2014; Travers, Tincani, & Lang, 2014), despite the absence of any compelling new evidence to support its efficacy (Schlosser et al., 2014).

The following exercise is based on a process of critical thinking and presents an opportunity to apply some questions to a brief article that may help you gain some insight into the FC controversy. It consists of using *argument analysis skills* as described by Browne and Keeley (2015). The questions and argument analysis process will help guide your interpretation and evaluation of a case study by Shane and Kearns (1994). This study of FC was designed to determine if the client was the actual source of his typed responses to an examiner's questions or if the facilitator was inadvertently guiding the client and, thus, the real source of the responses. In effect, this was a test to determine who was doing the "talking"—the client or the facilitator?

Step 1—Do you have biases or assumptions about FC?

In order to keep our exercise manageable, we will only apply a subset of the critical thinking questions that relate to interpretation and evaluation (see Figure 3–1). First, as a critical thinker, it is imperative that you understand what your biases and assumptions are about FC. This is an important starting point because if you already have a strong opinion—either positive or negative—about a treatment approach before you begin looking at the evidence, then you need to be aware that this might shape your analysis of the evidence. For example, if you have a positive view, and if the evidence is also positive, you may be more likely to look at the findings favorably, no matter what the quality of the study may or may not be. On the other hand, if you have a negative view, you may look at the same evidence and view it unfavorably, even if the quality of the study was relatively good. Therefore, your self-knowledge of your views beforehand will be important so that you can monitor how much this knowledge might be influencing your thinking, and whether or not you are being fair-minded as you move to your final conclusion. Take a moment right now and jot down what it is you know about FC.

Step 2—Read the research.

Once you have recorded your thoughts on FC, you will need to access and read the original article by Shane and Kearns (1994)—the complete reference is provided for you at the end of this exercise. This is the case we will use for practicing the critical thinking skills of argument analysis.

Step 3—Interpretation (Frame the argument)

Interpretation is the first phase of argument analysis. Your goal is to try to understand an author's argument in terms of its issue, conclusion, and reasons. This is an important starting point because if you cannot accurately frame the author's argument, you will either be unable to evaluate the argument because you realize you don't understand what the author's argument is or if you framed it inaccurately, you will evaluate an argument, but not the one the author intended. To begin the interpretation phase of your analysis of Shane and Kearns (1994), consider the following questions: (1) What is the issue for the Shane and Kearns study? (2) What was their conclusion? And (3) what were their reasons for arriving at this conclusion? Try addressing these questions on your own first, before reading the following sections.

What is the issue for the Shane and Kearns study? An issue is the question or controversy that is under consideration (Browne & Keeley, 2015) in an argument. The issue for a research study is usually straightforward and easy to find because it will usually be the specific purpose for the study, which you can locate in the Abstract or Introduction sections of a journal article. The issue for the Shane and Kearns study was to determine the extent to which the individual (DM), who was believed to communicate via a facilitator, was actually generating his own messages.

What was their conclusion? The conclusion is the "bottom line"; it's what the author of an argument wants you to believe or do relative to the issue (Browne & Keeley, 2015). The conclusion of a research study is also straightforward and easy to find in a research report. It is typically the investigator's interpretation of the study's results and it can usually be found in the Abstract or Conclusion sections of a journal article. On the basis of the results of their study, Shane and Kearns (1994) concluded that the facilitator was strongly influencing the messages produced by DM.

What were their reasons for arriving at this conclusion? Reasons are the basis for believing or justifying a conclusion (Browne & Keeley, 2015). Identifying the reasons is an important step in critical thinking. First, they are essential if you want to be able to evaluate the credibility of a conclusion. And it is important to appreciate that not all reasons are good reasons; some are better than others. Second, the reasons may provide an opportunity for you to be open to another person's views. For example, if the author's reasons are sufficiently convincing in support for their conclusion, then you may decide that this conclusion is one worth considering especially if it was counter to your original view on the issue. The reasons are easy to find in a research study because they are typically found in the Results section, and abbreviated versions of those reasons can also be located in the Abstract and Discussion sections. There were several reasons for Shane and Kearns's (1994) conclusion that are found on pages 51 and 52 of their report. As you will have read, Shane and Kearns designed four basic tasks that required DM to type his answer to the investigator's questions while DM was being supported by the facilitator. Each task was divided into two conditions that were referred to as "shared" and "unshared." During the shared condition, both DM and the facilitator were presented with the same information before DM was asked to respond to a question. For example, when DM was asked to label a picture, in the shared condition, both DM and the facilitator were shown the same picture (e.g., a radio). During the unshared condition, DM was asked to label a picture that was different from the one the facilitator saw. The results of these tasks and their two conditions are summarized by Shane and Kearns in Table 1 on page 51 of the article.

As you can see, when both DM and the facilitator shared the same information, DM responded to the question correctly. That is, during the shared picture labeling task, DM labeled the picture correctly when he typed his response with the support of the facilitator. In comparison, when DM and the facilitator unwittingly did not share the same information, DM's response was incorrect. For example, when DM was shown a picture of a radio and the facilitator was shown a picture of a knife, DM's typed response with the support of the facilitator was based on the picture the facilitator was shown (e.g., knife) and not the picture DM was shown (e.g., radio). The results as summarized in Table 1 are clear. For the shared condition, DM's responses were always correct or accurate. For the unshared condition, DM's responses were always incorrect or unintelligible. Based on these reasons, would you agree with Shane and Kearns' (1994) conclusion that it appeared that the facilitator was strongly influencing the messages produced by DM?

Step 4—Evaluation

Evaluation is the second phase of argument analysis. Your goal is to determine how acceptable you believe the author's conclusion is in view of the quality of the reasons provided to support it. One objective of this phase is to examine how credible you believe the reasons are that have been offered in support of the conclusion. For instance, if the reasons appear to have come from a high-quality source of information, such as a well-designed research study, you might be more readily convinced by the reasons. On the other hand, if the reasons came from a less certain source, such as a story that was found at a website, you might not be as convinced. On the basis of your evaluation, you will then attempt to arrive at a conclusion of your own about the credibility of the author's claim. Remember you may also want to consider to what extent your own biases and assumptions about the issue might be influencing your evaluation.

Now let's try to evaluate the credibility of the reasons that Shane and Kearns (1994) provided to support the conclusion of their study. For a research study, the credibility of the reasons relies heavily on the methods the authors used to obtain their results. For any research study, there are some basic questions that you can ask when you look at the Methods section. For example, how many participants contributed to the results of the study—a few or many? Look at the procedures for obtaining the findings that led to the results; do they appear to be biased in any way? How about the measures that were used to obtain the results; do they appear trustworthy and appropriate to the study's questions? These are just a few of the questions that can be posed to evaluate the credibility of a research study's results. Sometimes it helps to ask these questions from an alternative perspective, as if you were someone who was unsympathetic to the study's question but at the same time willing to be reasonable and practical. Take a look at Shane and Kearns' study and determine if you have any questions or concerns about how they obtained their results. Here are some of the questions you might ask when you look at the Methods section of Shane and Kearns' (1994) study: (1) Were one individual and facilitator sufficient to address the study's issue? And for that matter, were DM and his facilitator the most appropriate for this study's question? (2) Was the setting for conducting the study appropriate for the test? (3) Were the testing procedures appropriate for addressing the issue? And (4) how were the test responses scored?

Were one individual and facilitator sufficient to address the study's issue? There was only one pair of participants—DM and his facilitator. Obviously, one pair only for addressing the issue is limiting because they may be unique in unknown ways, and thus, they may not be a fair test of FC. However, as a careful reading reveals, this study was done under unique circumstances because it was conducted at the request of a local district attorney. Therefore, the legal context of this study limited the test to one pair only. That said, it should be noted that more recently, Schlosser et al. (2014) reviewed 31 studies that attempted to address similar issues to the one carried out by Shane and Kearns, and all of the studies concluded that "messages generated through [facilitated communication] are authored by facilitators rather than the individuals with disabilities" (p. 359). Based on the description of DM, he appeared to be the type of person for whom FC is usually recommended (cf. Biklen, 1992). In addition, his facilitator had successfully completed training in FC at a well-known facility at Syracuse University. She had also worked with DM for several years and reportedly had a good rapport with him. In contrast, if DM and the facilitator had only met for the first time for this study, we might be concerned that the absence of a good client–clinician relationship was interfering with the effectiveness of FC. But that did not appear to be a concern for this study.

Was the setting for conducting the study appropriate for the test? The testing was conducted in a room at the sheltered workshop where DM had worked for 4 years. The same equipment that DM and the facilitator had used for communicating was used for obtaining DM's responses during the tasks. It seems reasonable to assume that this would be a comfortable testing situation for DM and his facilitator.

Were the testing procedures appropriate for addressing the issue? The tasks designed to address the study's question appeared to be straightforward. They included labeling everyday pictures, answering questions related to pictures, naming everyday objects, and describing simple but unique events (e.g., blowing out a birthday candle). These seem like tasks that would be appropriate for someone with DM's presumed capabilities and life experiences. In contrast, if the tasks had been challenging or high level, we might be concerned that the testing procedures were biased against DM's ability to perform well with FC.

How were the test responses scored? DM's typed responses were printed in unmodified form and then scored after the testing had occurred, as correct or incorrect according to criteria that appeared to be reasonably flexible (e.g., words that contained 50% or more correct letters were scored correct). The authors of the study scored DM's responses independently and comparisons for each of their scored items showed they were in 100% agreement with each other. Thus, there doesn't appear to be any aspect of the scoring procedures that was inappropriate or weighted against DM receiving a good score. However, we might have preferred that "blind" scorers who were unaware of the study's purpose had scored the responses rather than the study's authors.

Step 5—What do you think?

This exercise provided you with an opportunity to apply some of the argument analysis skills described by Browne and Keeley (2015) to a case study presented by Shane and Kearns (1994). Based on this opportunity, what would you conclude about the claim of FC proponents that their approach has the potential to reveal undocumented literacy skills and thinking abilities of people with autism spectrum disorder (ASD) (e.g., Biklen, 1992)? Did Shane and Kearns' test of this claim raise questions for you about the credibility of FC? If it did, why do you think many practitioners continue to be trained in FC and provide it to people with ASD? What would you do as a future practitioner if you were to encounter a helping professional who advocated using FC with her clients? These are difficult questions that don't have easy answers. But they are important questions especially if you believe that as a helping professional, it is your responsibility to make the best possible decisions for people who seek your guidance and that you believe those decisions should be based on the best possible evidence that was examined by asking the right questions with an open- and fair-minded attitude. If there is one lesson we might learn from the FC controversy, it is the importance of making choices for our clients that are based on evidence-related hope rather than wishful thinking or false hope.

If you still have questions, then that's probably a good start! Perhaps this will prompt you to investigate the basis for your treatment decisions in the future. And that you are beginning to develop an appreciation for taking responsibility for understanding why you believe what you believe, and that it is not just what you think that matters when it comes to clinical decision making, but how you think.

Additional Critical Thinking Exercise
The following is a suggested reading that instructors might consider for further discussion of the FC controversy and helping students to appreciate the importance of critical thinking and a questioning approach to treatment claims.

Lilienfeld, S. O., Marshall, J., Todd, J. T., & Shane, H. C. (2014). The persistence of fad interventions in the face of negative scientific evidence: Facilitated communication for autism as a case example. *Evidence-Based Communication Assessment and Intervention, 8*, 62–101. doi:10.1080/17489539.2014.976332

Lilienfeld et al. (2014) have written a thorough and in-depth examination of fad interventions that persist even in the face of negative evidence with a focus on facilitated communication. Some questions that might guide a class discussion include the following:

1. Early in their paper, Lilienfeld et al. suggest three reasons for why the "tenacity of FC" is of importance to us. What are these reasons? What do you think of these reasons; do they seem like good ones?
2. Lilienfeld et al. provide a history of FC. The first part describes its "spectacular rise." What were some of the factors that contributed to its rise? Which of these stand out for you and why? Are you aware of any recent treatments (e.g., medical, drugs) or health-related products (e.g., diets, vitamins, etc.) that appear to have similar factors that are influencing how we (the public) regard them?
3. Scientific discrediting of FC was based on two methods described on p. 68. What were they? Have you heard of these kinds of scientific methods for testing treatments before? Do these methods as a means for objectively assessing a treatment's effectiveness seem credible to you, and why or why not?
4. Lilienfeld et al. describe how FC was discredited and the scientific consensus that emerged. Then the response from the FC proponents is described. Given these two sides to the story, what do you think?
5. Lilienfeld et al. attempt to document the "persistence" in use of FC via survey data and media coverage (pp. 71–76). What did you think of what they reported? Did they make their case?
6. They then go on to provide additional reasons that may be continuing to provide legitimacy to FC as a valid treatment—what were they (pp. 67–84)? Were you convinced?

7. Lilienfeld et al. provide various suggestions for why they believe FC has persisted on pages 85–89. What were these suggestions? Which ones stood out for you?

8. Finally, the authors conclude with various recommendations for how we might combat false treatments. What were these recommendations? And at the end of the day, do you think we as helping professionals should care about combating these false treatments? Maybe we should let our clients find their own way. We live in the information age; they'll find out eventually which treatments are bogus and which ones are real. Is it really our responsibility as helping professionals to know the difference?

Elements 2 and 3:
The Clinician, The Client

Chapter Outline

Learning Objectives

- The reader will learn how clinical experience and clinical expertise differ.
- The reader will learn about various characteristics of clinicians that facilitate change.
- The reader will learn about cultural sensitivity in different disciplines, including medicine, allied health, and communication sciences and disorders.
- The reader will learn about client/patient factors that may affect the clinical process.

The synthesis of being both caring and scientific may be one of the highest ideals for a clinician to achieve.

—Goldberg (1997, p. 313)

When it comes to clinical observation, we often think about the client/patient and the diagnosis. And yet, I am convinced that the journey toward becoming a master clinician has very little to do with diagnoses and everything to do with how we integrate our own personal experiences with those we observe. In this section, we delve into what characteristics make a "master" clinician and we explore literature about client/patient perspectives on the professionals with whom they interact. Also, we practice observing clinician behaviors. The aim is to work toward integrating what we know about ourselves with those features observed in master clinicians.

A developmental approach to achieving mastery in mental health counseling is put forward by Skovholt and Jennings (2005) in a special section of the *Journal of Mental Health Counseling* on master therapists. These authors, having conducted considerable research on what characteristics appear to identify expertise in clinicians, suggest there are four elements that appear to facilitate the evolution from beginning therapist to expert. They term these *signposts*, documenting how the process of becoming an expert clinician parallels the stages we progress through in life, and for beginning clinicians, the work starts with doing what you know and have skill with while learning the therapeutic process. As one moves along the path toward mastery, one must have the will to continue to learn, work in an environment that fosters and supports growth, and actively engage in reflection.

The Master Clinician

If we were to ask clients or patients what characteristics describe their "best" service providers, we likely would get a different answer from each of them depending, of course, on their experiences, the contexts of those experiences, and the outcomes. The concept of an "expert" or "master" clinician has been studied in a number of fields, with particular scrutiny in mental health counseling. Jennings, Goh, Skovholt, Hanson, and Banerjee-Stevens (2003) outline five factors that appear to be related to expertise in mental health counseling. These factors include experience, characteristics, openness to change/experience, cultural competence, and tolerance for ambiguity. A brief discussion of these factors is presented here to help frame our understanding of clinical expertise.

Clinical Experience

Experience is sometimes believed to be the most important factor associated with expertise or mastery in the clinical world. In fact, Jennings, Hanson, Skovholt, and Grier (2005) point out that the word *expert* is derived from the Latin word for experience, thus the conception that a master is one who has formed an expertise on the basis of experience. Some research supports this perspective. For example, Jennings et al. (2005) describe work involving different types of tasks and learners in a variety of fields, showing that, often, expertise or a capacity to excel at a particular set of tasks can be developed through prolonged study, practice, and experience. At the same time, other research on the role of experience in determining clinical outcomes does not always support the supposition that experience leads to expert knowledge and skill (e.g., Kivighlan & Quigley, 1991; Stein & Lambert, 1995). In a review of expertise in nursing, McHugh and Lake (2010) state that "Experience is a necessary but not sufficient condition for expertise . . ." (p. 278). And, although a fair amount of support does exist for a large contribution of experience to level of expertise, other factors are related to the level of proficiency or expertise exhibited by nurses.

Jennings et al. (2003) assert that, while experience allows clinicians to conceptualize the therapeutic process in more sophisticated ways, it does not always guarantee successful outcomes. What experienced clinicians demonstrate more so than do inexperienced clinicians is the ability to draw on a well-established store of knowledge and implement adaptations to treatment while in the process of conducting therapy (Martin, Slemon, Hiebert, Hallman, & Cummings, 1989; Orlinsky et al., 1999). Leonard and Swap (2005) refer to this as having "deep smarts," possessing not only vast knowledge but also experience with using both system-level and individual-level components in quick decision making. So, we recognize that experience plays a substantial role in the development of expertise, but it is just one factor related to mastery.

The role of experience in the development of a master clinician in CSD has not been adequately researched. In 1993, the American Speech-Language-Hearing Association (ASHA) produced a monograph detailing research on *Language Interactions in Clinical and Educational Settings*. A major thrust of this work included the argument that the assessment of elements of speech and language, when examined in isolation, holds little merit for helping us understand the nature of communication impairments (Damico, 1993). At that time, Damico (1993) referred to "failures" experienced by all clinicians—failures that reflected the difficulty the profession had with a "mismatch between professional expectations and professional expertise" (p. 92). Damico maintained that our development of clinical expertise must advance to embrace a "synergistic orientation" in which speech and language behavior is regarded in context, leading to the use of "more 'interactive,' 'naturalistic,' and 'socially valid' methods of treatment" (p. 95). Much of the content of this book examines the occurrence or implementation of these very features, for example, client-/patient-centered practice (i.e., interaction), delivery in naturalistic environments (naturalistic), and the consideration of sociocultural influences (socially valid).

As an observer of clinical interactions, you have begun your own process of obtaining clinical experience. On the surface, the "act" of observing seems passive, and yet, with the identification of specific goals and strategies for gleaning information to help you achieve the goals, your observational work becomes active. And, because you seek out different observation opportunities, your clinical experience naturally expands. Take, for example, the opportunity to observe an interprofessional team conducting a developmental evaluation of a 30-month-old child. Team members invite you to sit in on the assessment, which is conducted with a developmental pediatrician, a speech-language pathologist (SLP), a social worker, a physical therapist, and the child's mother and grandmother—all in the room with the youngster. Rather than watching a process unfold on a screen or through an observation window, you are able to observe firsthand how the child responds differently to his mother and grandmother than he does to the professionals. You can hear the child humming softly while wandering around the room gazing at the light fixtures and electrical outlets. Suddenly, you find yourself in a position to help redirect the child away from the sink in the corner of the room, and your role as observer has changed. Now, you are a participant observer; you feel an energy you wouldn't otherwise have felt, and the information you are collecting involves active experience. That experience includes direct contact with the client/patient, his family members, and the team and becomes a part of your foundation in clinical work.

Clinical Expertise

How is expertise defined? Expertise is one of the three components of evidence-based practice, along with client/patient preferences and values and scientific evidence. In health-related fields, clinical expertise can be taken for granted. That is, if one has the credentials for audiology, speech-language pathology, nursing, medicine, etc., it is expected that the practitioner has the expertise. In reality, this is not always the case, as students' and professionals' access to training programs, opportunities for experience, the availability of repeated practice, and constructive feedback differ. And, perspectives on what constitutes mastery or expertise also differ. For example, in surgical medicine, expertise might be defined as having particular manual skill in the operating room; or, in the lab, expert pathologists might make use of specific visual strategies. Most recent work on expertise in medicine now recognizes that it involves much more than "know-how" or isolated skills (e.g., Jaarsma, Jarodzka, Nap, van Merriënboer, & Boshuizen, 2015; Kirkman, 2013). A model of "expert performance with deliberate practice" (Ericsson, 2015) has been advocated for facilitating physician expertise (Sklar, 2015). The model of expert performance with deliberate practice uses the identification of "reproducibly superior performance" that can be standardized and then taught through deliberate practice, which involves specially designed tasks that are practiced by an individual under the direction of a coach or teacher (Ericsson, 2015). Although such an approach might be suitable for certain areas of medicine, it does not always lend itself to fostering expertise development when objective measurement of "reproducible superior performance" may not be readily observable. For example, certain types of therapy (e.g., psychotherapy and speech and language therapy) make use of clinical skills that cannot be objectively measured given all of the factors that make up a therapeutic encounter that cannot be controlled (e.g., client/patient response, and environmental). Thus, the expert performance-deliberate practice model may be applicable to CSD in that it reinforces the importance of deliberate practice, but it may not be a model for all aspects of the discipline. For students observing clinical work, deliberate practice might mean specific activities aimed at practicing the skill of identifying important data to collect or using objective language in clinical descriptions. More importantly, observation must include the recognition that clinical expertise not only involves extensive "practice," it also reflects individual characteristics of the practitioner and the impact of contextual factors, for example, the work environment, including coworkers (e.g., McHugh & Lake, 2010).

One of the only studies of clinical expertise identified that includes CSD professionals (SLPs) is an examination of the decision-making skills of novice, intermediate, and expert clinicians from a variety of disciplines involved with pediatric rehabilitation (King et al., 2007). After determining the level of expertise (i.e., novice, intermediate, expert) using a method involving peer, self, and parent measures, the authors conducted two separate studies involving interviews with a total of 24 professionals, including occupational therapists (10), physical therapists (7), SLPs (4), behavior therapists (2), and recreation therapists (1). In the first interview, the therapists were asked to reflect on one or two "critical" clinical events (positive or negative) that affected their thinking. In the second interview, the therapists were asked to "think aloud" about their decision making while viewing a videotape of themselves with a client. Analyses of the interviews were organized around particular changes that took place in three areas: (1) content knowledge ("changes in approaches and expectations with developing expertise"), (2) self-knowledge, and (3) procedural knowledge ("changes in therapeutic strategies").

The most central content knowledge theme is one of an evolving approach to treatment that the authors describe as "A supportive, educational, holistic, functional and strengths-based approach" (King et al., 2007, p. 223). The course clinicians describe is one of moving away from seeing themselves as a "fixer" of the problem to one of a facilitator, who identifies functional goals, is more inclusive of family, and is less judgmental. The second area of change, self-knowledge, is described by the authors as "heightened humility, yet increased self-confidence" (King et al., 2007, p. 229). In this process, clinicians report using more self-assessment and forming more realistic expectations. They also acquire greater trust in the therapy process and a self-confidence that allows them to admit when they might not know the answer. This confidence is also shown in a level of comfort working with a diversity of families. Finally, the third area of change, procedural knowledge, is marked by "The use of principles of change, and enabling and customizing strategies" (King et al., 2007, p. 229). Principles of change revolve around making the therapeutic process more effective, underlined by three tenets: "(a) engage the client and family . . . (b) make therapy meaningful for the client . . . and (c) make the intervention more manageable . . ." (King et al., 2007, p. 230). For the goal of "engaging the client and family," expert clinicians use strategies of motivation and adaptation. According to King et al. (2007), these include such strategies as creating rapport, ensuring comfort and enjoyment, and making sure the child experiences success. Additionally, expert clinicians demonstrate the ability to make adjustments to treatment in order to maximize the client's growth (e.g., providing opportunities that push the client to the next level without creating frustration or failure). Most of the clinicians in the study exhibited strategies that work to match the session expectations with the client's skills, such as obtaining feedback and pacing the session appropriately.

"Making therapy meaningful" (the second outcome goal) is accomplished with strategies that entail consistency, unity, and a sound rationale ("It makes sense."). These strategies make use of clarification, observation, and explanation. In individualizing therapy, expert and intermediate clinicians are more likely to employ tactics that adjust goals, objectives, and/or planning to customize the intervention. For example, these types of clinicians address priorities with family and in therapy and show skill with modifying intervention procedures to best meet the client's needs.

"Manageability," fostering the client's sense of control, is accomplished with the types of strategies that encourage decision making in the client and family and make sure the intervention is appropriate and possible. Such tactics might include guiding problem solving, making it so the client and/or family takes the lead in therapy, and providing information that helps with decision making. Strategies for making therapy "work" for individual clients and their families are utilized by all levels of therapists. Novice, as well as intermediate and expert, therapists demonstrate the ability to set realistic goals, provide choices of activities for clients, and divide complex tasks into manageable pieces. On the other hand, only experts are observed to make certain therapy moves at a comfortable pace.

In brief, the King et al. (2007) study shows a developmental process toward a clinician with skill at adapting strategies to best facilitate change and positive outcomes. These authors note that their findings are similar, in many ways, to those of others (e.g., Skovholt, Jennings, & Mullenbach, 2004) and that expertise involves evolution, particularly with respect to knowledge about content, self, and process. When it comes to content, expert therapists hold a broader and deeper knowledge base that supports them in seeing "the big picture" and incorporating multiple perspectives into the therapeutic process. This allows them to be more open minded and holistic in their approach. Advanced self-awareness is manifested in expert clinicians as a general level of comfort with the therapeutic relationship and process of intervention. Increased confidence and humility and "realistic and refined expectations" are all indicators of expert self-knowledge. Finally, procedural knowledge advances greatly from novice to expert. Specifically, King et al. note areas in which expert clinicians reveal their sophistication with procedures:

> . . . (a) Their ability to manage the context of the intervention in order to maximize the likelihood of change, (b) their ability to work on various short-, mid-, and longer-term goals simultaneously, and (c) their flexible and creative use of specific strategies to empower clients and customize intervention efforts. (p. 234)

In describing the strategies used by therapists in pediatric rehabilitation disciplines, the authors remind the reader that the essence of the expert clinician is one in which all aspects of treatment (including relationships with all stakeholders) are managed skillfully over the course of the therapeutic process. The facets comprising that skillful manager are contemplated in the following section on "Clinician Characteristics."

Clinician Characteristics

A considerable amount of support has been amassed for the understanding that the clinician represents the most critical factor related to success in therapy (Baldwin & Imel, 2013). In particular, the mental health counseling and psychotherapy literature has identified specific characteristics that are associated with more effective clinicians. These include the ability to establish a better partnership (Baldwin, Wampold, & Imel, 2007), highly developed interpersonal skills (Anderson, Ogles, Patterson, Lambert, & Vermeersch, 2009), and the ability to foster a relationship that allows for emotional exploration (Laska, Smith, Wislocki, Minami, & Wampold, 2013). Other factors identified by Jennings et al. (2003) include the characteristics of "experts" or master clinicians. These authors point out that research from such disparate fields as business, physics, and psychotherapy has identified a variety of cognitive strengths observed in experts. Missing from past lists of "expert skills," however, are those skills related to emotion and relationship building. Skovholt and Jennings (2004) provide a summary of research investigating the characteristics of master therapists, concluding that a more comprehensive model of expertise in mental health counseling includes advanced skill in cognitive, emotional, and relational domains. What does it mean to have advanced skill in the cognitive domain? Skovholt (2005) suggests that one must have ". . . an ability to flexibly embrace complex ambiguity, accumulate wisdom, understand the human condition, and make learning a lifelong adventure" (p. 83). Skill in the emotional domain, Skovholt submits, includes the ". . . acceptance of self, genuine humility, self-awareness, a willingness to grow and gain competence, a passion for life, quiet strength, and an appreciation for life in the moment" (p. 83). And, importantly, one with astute relational expertise demonstrates ". . . the ability to intensively engage with others, keen interpersonal perception, being led by the well-being of the client, expressing compassion within limits, making accurate judgements, and remaining open to learning from others" (p. 83).

An Exercise on Cognitive, Emotional, and Relational Domains
Using the descriptions provided above, describe yourself in terms of cognitive, emotional, and relational skills. Where do you see your strengths? Where do you see your needs? How might you work to improve in all domains, and what would that look like in clinical practice?

As stated, research substantiates the vital role of the clinician in positive outcomes in mental health counseling. What about other disciplines? Following are brief descriptions of some of the research that has been conducted on clinician characteristics. These particular studies are highlighted because they provide differing perspectives on what constitutes a "good" or "ideal" practitioner and the results highlight some of the fundamentals espoused in this text (e.g., reflection and openness to experience).

Schattner, Rudin, and Jellin (2004) conducted one of the first studies to examine characteristics of "good" physicians in populations of both hospitalized and clinic patients. Using a questionnaire in which patients were asked to rank qualities of "good" physicians, the authors obtained lists of the most desirable and least desirable physician attributes within three domains: (1) the domain of patient's autonomy and rights, (2) the domain of professional expertise, and (3) the domain of humanism and support. In terms of priority with respect to which of these domains is endorsed most often, items within the professional expertise domain are identified more often than any of the other domains. Even though it is seen as the highest priority, when examining the "best" qualities of physicians, only two of the top eight qualities fall within that domain. Table 4–1 lists the top qualities and their respective domains endorsed by at least 25% of the patients in the Schattner et al. investigation. We see that the most frequently occurring domain is that of "patient rights and autonomy," as half of the top eight qualities come from that domain. The characteristic most frequently endorsed is that of "very experienced and professional," as 50% of all patients ranked this as a most desirable trait. The authors note that the findings are stable across other characteristics of the population studied, such as demographic or medical variables. The findings of this study are interesting in that they are not consistent with later research suggesting the importance of humanistic medicine (see Campos, 2005, for humanities and medicine). In summarizing, the authors claim, "The age of paternalism in medical care has come to an end. . . . Most patients want to be informed about their health care even if the news are bad . . . and to be involved with their care plans . . ." (p. 26).

A comparable study completed by Bendapudi, Berry, Frey, Turner Parish, and Rayburn (2006) examines patients' descriptions of their "best" and "worst" physician encounters in the Mayo Clinic system. Through transcription of the interviews and theme analysis, the authors identify seven features that appear to best define "ideal" physician characteristics. These are listed in Table 4–2.

Table 4–1. Most Desired Qualities of "Good" Physicians

Domain	Top qualities	Patients endorsed (%)
Professional expertise	Is very experienced and professional.	50
	Is current with new developments in medicine.	28
Patient's autonomy and rights	Provides clear explanation, elaborates on treatment options and possible adverse outcomes.	36
	Asks patient's opinion about what might be wrong.	29
	Tells whole truth about condition and treatment.	28
	Finds out what is important to patient and takes into consideration patient preferences.	25
Humanism and support	Shows patience and devotes enough time.	38
	Is very attentive.	30

Source: Adapted from Schattner, Rudin, and Jellin (2004).

Table 4–2. Ideal Physician Behaviors and Definitions

Ideal physician behaviors	Definitions
Confident	The doctor's assured manner engenders trust. The doctor's confidence gives me confidence.
Empathetic	The doctor tries to understand what I am feeling and experiencing, physically, emotionally, and communicates that understanding to me.
Humane	The doctor is caring, compassionate, and kind.
Personal	The doctor is interested in me more than just as a patient, interacts with me, and remembers me as an individual.
Forthright	The doctor tells me what I need to know in plain language and in a forthright manner.
Respectful	The doctor takes my input seriously and works with me.
Thorough	The doctor is conscientious and persistent.

Source: Adapted from Bendapudi, Berry, Frey, Turner Parish, and Rayburn (2006).

Similar to the findings of Schattner et al. (2004), Bendapudi et al. report that the ideal characteristics of physicians are those that preserve the patient's autonomy and rights (e.g., "The doctor takes my input seriously . . . ," "The doctor tells me what I need to know . . .") and represent a humanistic approach ("The doctor tries to understand what I am feeling and experiencing . . . and communicates that understanding to me."). Unlike Schattner et al., however, the results of the interviews with the Mayo Clinic patients reveal little in the way of professional expertise as being a feature of the "ideal" physician. Closest to this might be comments provided by the interviewees that reflected physician confidence and persistence. For example, Bendapudi et al. provide sample quotes supporting these attributes:

> You could tell by his attitude that he was very strong, very positive, very confident that he could help me. (p. 340)

> My cardiac surgeon explained everything very well. The explanation was very thorough. He was very concerned about my recovery after the surgery. (p. 340)

In reflecting on the nature of the comments gathered from patients and the rarity of remarks involving physician expertise, the authors state that true observation of the technical or functional capabilities of physicians is often hard to obtain. Patients may not know what to look for or may not have an opportunity to observe actual skill. Therefore, they rely on what they are able to observe—typically the behavior of the physician. As Bendapudi et al. (2006) express, "Patients can sense if the physician is rushed, preoccupied, tired, aloof, disinterested, or alarmed just as they can sense a physician's genuine interest, compassion, calmness and confidence" (p. 341). The authors offer a model in which patients are "detectives" looking for "clues" to render a determination of the quality of their physician. The "clues" that patients pay attention to fall into three categories, which the authors term "functional" clues—reflecting technical skills; "mechanic" clues—material characteristics (e.g., sights, sounds, environmental); and "humanic"—the behaviors and appearance of the physician. At the end of the chapter is an exercise designed to help you recognize clinical behaviors that are consistent with those of the "ideal" physician, as constructed by Bendapudi et al.

In a more recent study of desirable characteristics of both nurses and doctors, Haron and Tran (2014) interviewed inpatients in a mental health hospital. Content analyses of interviews reveal similar themes for both sets of professionals, although slight differences are observed. The top five desirable characteristics of nurses include encouraging, compassionate, available, understanding, and cooperative. For doctors, the top five are supportive, available, cooperative, humane, and caring. In terms of overall findings, the authors identify three primary expectations expressed by all patients, regardless of health status. Both doctors and nurses are expected to (1) treat the patient with respect, as a whole person, not just a disease, illness, or diagnosis; (2) involve the patient in decision making; and (3) provide emotional support. In summary, the researchers stress that the establishment of a "quality relationship" with health care providers is what patients perceived as the most important component of what makes a good doctor or nurse. What is interesting about these findings is that patients did not express a desire for either nurses or doctors to bring disciplinary expertise to the interaction. This may reflect the nature of the population studied in the Haron and Tran study. As hospitalized patients with significant mental health disorder, this population may perceive the roles of the nurse and doctor differently than do outpatient populations.

Table 4–3. Domains of Master Genetic Counselor Characteristics

Domain	Top characteristics
Defining Traits and Attitudes	Insatiable curiosity, lifelong learning, deep knowledge
	Deep empathetic understanding
	Self-reflection
Influences on Development	Influence from colleagues
	Learning from patients
	"Infectious excitement," impact of mentoring
Process of Development	Development occurs over time and experience
	Quality of experience over quantity of experience
Impact of the "Person"	Realistic expectations of oneself
	One's personality is one's counseling style
	Use of self, genuine, comfortable in one's own skin
Distinctive Practice	Being fully present and engaged
	Attunement to the multiple levels of the genetic counseling process
Inspirations	Patience
	Deep personal meaning from the work
Emotional Impact	Loss, sadness, helplessness, communicating bad news

Source: Adapted from Miranda, Veatch, Martyr, and LeRoy (2016).

A recent study of genetic counselors identifies several characteristics of those deemed "expert" by their colleagues (Miranda, Veatch, Martyr, & LeRoy, 2016). Using a qualitative design, the authors interviewed 15 active genetic counselors who were identified by their peers as "exemplary" professionals. Data analysis reveals seven domains that include 33 different categories. Table 4–3 lists the different domains into which participant responses were coded. The most often endorsed traits and attitudes include lifelong learning, expression of empathy, and self-reflection. Genetic counselors regard their patients as inspirational and of value in their own development as professionals. Echoed in these findings are the key areas identified by Skovholt (2005)—cognitive, emotional, and relational—and the processes we have been discussing—being open to continue learning and self-reflection.

A look at the literature on clinician characteristics and outcomes in the area of oncology reveals a number of attributes that are similar to those we have thus far reviewed (De Vries et al., 2014). Observations made by these authors include the following: those physicians who demonstrate empathy use an approach to care that is considered socioemotional and patient centered (in particular including the patient in decision making) and those who have received training in communication appear to have a positive impact on communicative effectiveness and/or patient outcome. The authors note that measures of patient experience, such as how consistently patients stick to a treatment plan, whether or not they believe in their ability to succeed (self-efficacy), or overall satisfaction, are related to the working relationship or the therapeutic alliance between the patient and the practitioner. The concept of a "therapeutic alliance," a fundamental tenet of clinical psychology, has implications for speech, language, swallowing, and hearing treatment (see Hooper, 1996; Manning, 2010; Millard & Cook, 2010). We will return to this principle in our discussion of the client–/patient–clinician relationship in Chapter 5.

In a departure from the health disciplines, findings from research in the area of career counseling can inform our understanding of effective practitioner characteristics. Whiston, Rossier, and Hernandez Barón (2016) identify important features of career counselors that appear to positively influence the process of counseling in career decision making. Specifically, their review of the literature indicates that a "working alliance" is fostered when the counselor establishes positive rapport with the client at the outset (Elad-Strenger & Littman-Ovadia (2012) and is perceived as empathetic and uses self-disclosure (Multon, Ellis-Kalton, Heppner, & Gysbers, 2003). They stress that a strong working alliance is focused on mutual goals, tasks, and the counselor–client bond (Masdonati, Perdrix, Massoudi, & Rossier, 2014). The best predictor of success for the process of career counseling is found to be the client's view of the working relationship (Elliott, Bohart, Watson, & Greenberg, 2011). The implications of this work for CSD professionals is that the development of a bond between the client/patient and the clinician is essential to the process of change, and the burden of initiating and maintaining that relationship falls on the professional.

Clinician characteristics have not been examined with any depth in the CSD discipline. Early research, using clinical supervisors' ratings of student clinician behaviors, shows three factors that appear most influential in the process of therapy (Oratio, 1976, 1980). In order of significance, these factors are "interpersonal relationship," "technical skills," and "target behavior." Included within the realm of interpersonal are behaviors such as showing respect, leaving time for responses, and accepting the client. Technical skills are behaviors such as those that maximize the use of target responses, modify treatment programming in response to client behaviors, and reinforce client approximations of the intended behavior. Target behavior includes behaviors of the clinician directed at client responses, including appropriate feedback and encouraging client self-correction and carryover. Oratio suggests that interpersonal skills in clinicians play a substantial role in the success of therapy.

As previously mentioned, Goldberg (1997) proposes that master SLPs (and I would add audiologists) embody the concept of "compassionate scientists," the definition of which is ". . . individuals who intensely care for the well-being of their clients, and endeavor to meet their needs in the most effective scientific manner" (p. 313). And, although the construct of a compassionate scientist and the characteristics associated with a master clinician that Goldberg proposes are not based on the results of an empirical study, they serve as a foundation for examining what makes a "good clinician." For the purposes of learning about clinician behavior through observation, we will focus on the six critical characteristics described in Table 4–4.

Table 4–4. Six Critical Characteristics of Master CSD Clinicians

Characteristic	Description
Facilitator	Someone who provides the conditions necessary for a person to develop a new behavior, attitude, or learn new information.
Exquisite timing	Someone who knows when to present information and when to withhold it.
Contingency thinking	The ability to anticipate a client/patient response before it occurs and provide the most appropriate response to it.
Consistency	The use of consistent skills.
Concentration on acquisition tasks	Spending time on acquisition tasks, rather than retrieval, yields the greatest gains.
Focus	The ability to focus solely on the needs of the client, requiring preparation and subversion of one's own needs.

Source: Adapted from Goldberg (1997).

Facilitator

A facilitator is someone who makes it possible for something to change, or a new skill to develop, typically by making the change process easier. Some changes are easier to make happen than others. For audiologists, fitting a hearing aid that provides amplification and allows a person to participate more readily in everyday activities may be a relatively easy process or a very involved process, depending on the nature of the hearing loss, the individual being fitted, and the circumstances in which that person functions. In stuttering therapy, facilitating fluency with a client can be relatively easy, simply by engaging in one or more fluency facilitating activities, such as choral reading. More difficult, of course, is facilitating that client's fluency outside the therapy environment, in the "real world." There is no single list of "expert facilitator" skills. Facilitative skills that a master clinician might demonstrate include being flexible and setting up a therapeutic process that allows for practice, feedback, and success. While conducting clinical observations, you might find it most helpful to keep in mind that the clinician does not make the change happen, rather she or he creates the best context (including the environment, process, and relationship—essentially everything) for bringing that change about.

In your next observation, look for evidence of facilitation. How did the clinician help the client or make change happen?

Exquisite Timing

The master clinician knows when to present information and when to withhold it. She or he continually assesses the progression of therapy to determine when the client/patient may be ready for something more advanced or when it is time to reduce demands. Much of timing depends on the relationship between the clinician and the client/patient. A master clinician will have developed a therapeutic alliance with her or his clients/patients, one that is based on trust and a shared understanding of the goals and expectations. This foundation allows for an understanding of needs and capabilities on which the master clinician can capitalize, making use of the intuitive sense that has been developed over the course of the intervention process.

In your next observation, look for evidence of exquisite timing. Describe what happened.

Contingency Thinking

Contingency thinking is one of the hallmark features that distinguish an expert clinician from a novice one. According to Goldberg (1997), "Contingency thinking is the ability to anticipate a client's response before it occurs, and provide the most appropriate response to it" (p. 316). When observing a master clinician, one sees what appears to be a seamless process, something like a choreographed dance between the clinician and the client/patient. In reality, the clinician is always thinking, anticipating, creating alternatives (contingencies). This skill is one that really only comes about with considerable experience, much trial and error, and self-reflection—making sure one uses the less-than-successful experiences to improve oneself.

In your next observation, look for evidence of contingency thinking. How can you tell the clinician was relying on contingency thinking? Can you find an example in which contingency thinking might have changed the outcome?

Consistency

Goldberg maintains that the biggest difference between expert clinicians and beginning or less experienced ones is that master clinicians employ their knowledge and skills much more consistently than do novice clinicians. The value of this characteristic cannot be overstated. Remember, we are in the business of change. Without consistent practice, consistent expectations, and consistent feedback, behavior is not likely to change. Consistency is a bedrock of the therapeutic process and should be carried out in everything the clinician does.

In your next observation, look for evidence of clinician consistency. Describe what this looks like.

Concentration on Acquisition Tasks

Master clinicians spend substantial amounts of time on acquisition tasks. That is, our clients/patients are learning or relearning skills. On some level, their communication is not automatic; they are in the process of gaining some skill or other, which requires attention and practice. A tenet of intervention is the notion of generalization. It is not realistic for us to teach our clients/patients every single aspect of communication; rather we expect them to learn strategies or rules that can be generalized or carried over into new speech, language, hearing, or swallowing behaviors. Thus, considerable effort put into acquiring the rule or strategy pays off in the long run with transfer and generalization of the skill. This is manifested as concentration on acquisition tasks.

In your next observation, look for evidence of concentration on acquisition tasks. What is the effect of this strategy?

Focus

Just like consistency and concentration on acquisition tasks, the master clinician has the ability to maintain complete focus on the tasks at hand: facilitating change in her or his client/patient. To be focused on what will best help the client/patient meet her or his goals, the clinician must let go of self and external factors. As Goldberg (1997) quotes one master clinician, "When a client comes to see me, he is putting a tremendous amount of trust in me. That's a huge responsibility. Because of this, I owe the client my undivided attention for the entire 50 minute session" (p. 319). Thus, the characteristic of "focus" differs from that of "concentration on acquisition tasks" as it refers to the clinician's state of mind, rather than the spotlight of therapy.

In your next observation, look for evidence of focus.

Openness to Experience/Change

Openness to change or openness to experience is a feature that has been identified in the master clinician (Candlin, 2002). Openness to experience is considered to be related to critical thinking (Facione, Sanchez, Facione, & Gainen, 1995). Facione et al. (1995) suggest that openness to experience reflects a desire to find truth in a given situation, advanced problem solving, and open mindedness. It has been associated with curiosity (Gwyer, 1999; Resnik & Jensen, 2003), engaging a client/patient with an open mind (Conway, 1998), and being open to receiving feedback on one's own performance (Skovholt et al., 2004). Also, the successful use of critical thinking processes in clinical decision making is seen in individuals who are described as open minded (Chen, Hsu, Chang, & Lin, 2016). In their study of nurse practitioners, Chen et al. (2016) find that nurses using both analytical and intuitive thinking processes are more sophisticated decision makers, are holistic in their approach to care, and employ reflective practice more so than do less experienced nurses. In studying the factors related to these characteristics, the authors note that empathy and openness predict analytical ways of decision making.

Studies of clinical psychologists and psychotherapists affirm the importance of being open minded as a defining feature of master therapists (see Wampold, 2001, for a review). Jennings et al. (2008) investigate the characteristics that best identify the master mental health therapist in the United States and in Singapore. Their findings underscore the value of openness to experience as a distinguishing quality of master clinicians. In both studies, therapists identified by their peers as master clinicians point out the importance of being flexible in their approach to therapy, having curiosity and continuing interest in learning, and personal growth.

In a companion study to their work on decision-making skills in pediatric rehabilitation therapists (King et al., 2007), King et al. (2008) focus on features that distinguish expert pediatric rehabilitation therapists from those who may have experience but are not considered masters. Their definition of expertise incorporates knowledge, skills, and personal characteristics through demonstration of ". . . appropriate, exceptional, or adaptive performance or behaviour in response to a situation that contains a degree of unpredictability or uncertainty . . ." (King et al., 2008, p. 110). In other words, these authors contend that expertise is best observed when circumstances are not always guaranteed. In describing the features of expert therapists, King et al. (2008) turn to the literature that suggests motivation, openness to experience, and the complexity of prior clinical experiences as key indicators. The authors examine the characteristics in a total of 71 therapists from five disciplines, including SLPs, physical therapists, occupational therapists, behavior therapists, and recreational therapists. When evaluating the relative contribution to advancement along an expertise continuum, therapists who exhibit high motivation and a willingness to continue learning (open to experience) and have considerable experience working with a clientele that presents complex needs are those who appear to develop expertise in an accelerated fashion. I would suggest that these three components, motivation, openness to experience, and clinical experience with complex cases, interact in that a motivated clinician strives to learn and seek truth, which can be translated into having an open-minded attitude, an attitude that allows the clinician to take on complicated circumstances with confidence.

Tolerance for Ambiguity

We are learning that master clinicians across a range of health care disciplines possess certain characteristics that tend to be fairly consistent. Naturally, mastery of knowledge and skills critical to the profession are essential, yet we also see that highly respected expert clinicians also demonstrate ways of approaching circumstances with open mindedness, curiosity, and the desire to meet the needs of their clients/patients. Research in the medical field has looked at the notion of tolerance for ambiguity as critical to the development of a well-rounded physician. Caulfield, Andolsek, Grbic, and Roskovensky (2014) remind us that tolerance for ambiguity can be related to an individual's inclination to seek out new experiences, as past research has shown that lower tolerance for ambiguity is related to perceiving new or different experiences as "sources of threat" (Budner, 1962). Thus, practitioners who have lower levels of tolerance for ambiguity or uncertainty may experience greater stress or burnout (Cooke, Doust, & Steele, 2013), particularly in situations that may involve complex clients/patients. Furthermore, work by Wayne et al. (2011) reveals changes in level of tolerance and enthusiasm for working with underserved populations. That is, medical students at the beginning of their schooling show significantly greater levels of tolerance for ambiguity, along with more positive attitudes about the poor and underserved populations than do medical students at the point of graduation. These findings are consistent with other studies showing increasingly negative attitudes toward medically underserved populations (e.g., Crandall, Reboussin, Michielutte, Anthony, & Naughton, 2007) and overall declines in empathy through the course of medical school (Hojat et al., 2009; Newton, Barber, Clardy, Cleveland, & O'Sullivan, 2008). There may be a number of reasons for these trends, not the least of which is the speculation that as medical students advance toward "real-life" practice, they become more technology dependent, relying more heavily on computer-generated findings regarding diagnosis and technologically delimited answers about treatment (Hojat et al., 2009). Moreover, as medical students transition to becoming practicing physicians, the need to demonstrate expertise and capability may lead to more restricted and less risky ways of treating patients in order to maintain a certain confidence. These conclusions resonate with those on observation skills put forth in Chapter 1.

There has been some discussion in the literature as to whether tolerance for ambiguity is a fixed trait or one that may be malleable (Geller, Faden, & Levine, 1990). For our understanding of this characteristic, we use the following definition, offered by McLain, Keffalonitis, and Armani (2015), "Ambiguity tolerance is an individual's systematic, stable tendency to react to perceived ambiguity with greater or lesser intensity" (p. 2). What this implies is that a person's level of tolerance for uncertainty is most likely a stable trait, although it can be impacted considerably by context and perception. Why should we, as audiologists and SLPs, be concerned about the presence of ambiguity and our ability to tolerate it in CSD practice? Because we work with humans, and the essential function of communication, and human nature, will never be entirely predictable—that's why.

Cultural Sensitivity

Audiologists and SLPs are expected to be responsive to all clients and patients in ways that are respectful of their culture. Although we all strive to develop a level of cultural competence that matches this pursuit, "competence" may mean very different things to different practitioners, clients, patients, and others. Rather than attempting to know all aspects of all cultures with competence, I would suggest we work toward practicing with cultural sensitivity, seeing each of our clients/patients as possessing their own, unique culture. Using an individual approach relieves some of the pressure to learn all that there is about a culture and allows the clinician to develop an alliance with the client/patient that is based on respect and mutual understanding. Individuation is discussed further in the next section on Culturally Sensitive Practice in Medicine and Allied Health.

While this text prefers to use the term *cultural sensitivity*, much of the literature discusses cultural considerations from the perspective of a practitioner's competence or proficiency. With respect to the development of cultural proficiency, Wells (2000) presents a developmental model based on both cognitive and affective processes. She argues that it is not enough for an individual to become culturally aware, sensitive, and competent; rather, without institutional commitment and work, true cultural competence/proficiency will not be achieved. It is beyond this text to delve into the issues surrounding institutional practices, yet, it is important for students (and professionals) to be reminded that progress in cultural competence is dependent on both individual and organizational factors. Table 4–5 presents Wells' model of the cognitive and affective processes involved in the development of cultural competence. Initially, an individual may be culturally incompetent. That is, she or he lacks knowledge regarding the role that cultural influences have in clinical practice. Further along, the student begins to grasp certain aspects of culture and its interaction with the health environment, and this knowledge helps to formulate an awareness of "the cultural implications of health behavior" (p. 190). At this point, a student (or professional) possesses information that fosters recognition and, perhaps, appreciation but may not yet be translating that knowledge into practice. In order to move to the affective processes, Wells asserts that it is imperative that we come to understand how our own beliefs and thoughts are formed, through personal experiences and a powerful socialization process. Once that work is undertaken, we can move into making choices for our clients/patients that are culturally appropriate. At this point in the process, we are practicing with cultural competence, according to Wells. Proficiency, "integration of cultural competence into the culture of the organization and into professional practice," Wells maintains, does not occur without systemic change—within both the institution and the individuals committing to and mastering the cognitive and emotional facets of culturally sensitive practice (p. 192).

In Medicine and Allied Health

Described as "a tour de force—a compelling story about race, health and conquering inequality in medical care" (Ogletree, n.d.)[1], Augustus White's (2011) book, *Seeing Patients: Unconscious Bias in Health Care*, uses the author's own story to tell of the impact of belonging or not belonging to groups with or without access to quality health care. To practice culturally sensitive care, one must develop an awareness, which, White asserts ". . . helps to validate people who belong to groups other than our own, people who might otherwise be devalued

---

[1] http://www.hup.harvard.edu/catalog.php?isbn=9780674049055&content=reviews

Table 4–5. Model of Cultural Development

	Cognitive phase		Affective phase	
Cultural incompetence	**Cultural knowledge**	**Cultural awareness**	**Cultural sensitivity**	**Cultural competence**	**Cultural proficiency**
A lack of knowledge of the cultural implications of health behavior	Learning the elements of culture and their role in shaping and defining health behavior	Recognizing and understanding the cultural implications of health behavior	The integration of cultural knowledge and awareness into individual and institutional behavior	The routine application of culturally appropriate health care interventions and practices	The integration of cultural competence into the culture of the organization, and into professional practice, teaching, and research. Mastery of the cognitive and affective phases of cultural development.

Source: Adapted from Wells (2000).

or disregarded, even if subconsciously" (p. 262). Research has documented the existence of disparities in health care along a number of dimensions, including social factors (Marmot, 2005; Wilkinson & Marmot, 2003). Along with race, gender, religion, age, and other factors, poor socioeconomic circumstances or economic instability greatly impact the quantity and quality of health care obtained. As well, the presence of disability predicts reduced access and quality of services (World Health Organization, 2011). In these contexts, we know that implicit bias or stereotype plays a role (e.g., Johnson, Saha, Arboleaz, Beach, & Cooper, 2004). How do these dynamics operate in the clinical world? Using a social-cognitive psychology framework, Burgess et al. (2007) identify three pertinent findings from the research:

> . . . (1) health-care providers hold stereotypes—based on patient race, class, sex, and other characteristics[4–17]—that influence their interpretations of behaviors and symptoms, and their clinical decisions[17–25]; (2) application of such stereotypes frequently takes place outside conscious awareness[26–31]; and (3) providers interact less effectively with minority than with white patients.[32–37] (p. 882)[2]

Research verifies the stability of these findings and how difficult implicit biases are to change (Devine & Monteith, 1999; Kawakami, Dovidio, Moll, Hermsen, & Russin, 2000; Wilson, Lindsey, & Schooler, 2000). Rather than attempting to modify all that goes into the formation of such attitudes and beliefs (i.e., personal experiences and sociocultural influences), Burgess et al. (2007) recommend providing new experiences and strategies that work to shape new perspectives. Empirical studies have shown changes in mindsets around implicit bias through the use of individuation—the practice of viewing another as an individual with characteristics unique to that person, rather than as someone belonging to an "other" group, such as portrayed by White (Brewer, 1988; Fiske, Lin, & Neuberg, 1999). Such practice is focused on the elements contained in a model put forth by Burgess et al. and presented in Figure 4–1. The model identifies several areas, grouped into the categories of motivation, information, emotion, and orientation, in which research has shown positive impacts on reducing bias. First, one must have an internal motivation for responding without bias. Without such motivation, individual clinicians are not likely to change in their practice patterns. One way to do so might be to remind clinicians that their primary goal is to provide the best care possible for their clients/patients.

Second, providing practitioners with information on how bias is developed and reinforced, the history of bias in health care and how disparities in health care are enhanced through implicit bias can prompt active reflection on their own stereotypes and how they might play out in practice. The authors are quick to point out that the act of identifying bias is often associated with negative

---

[2] Footnoted citations can be found in original.

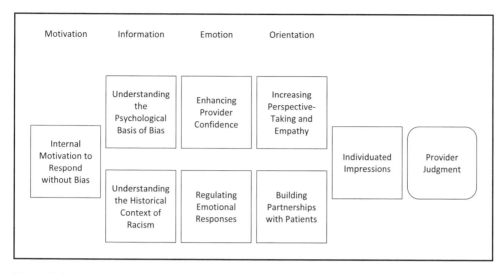

Figure 4–1. Conceptual framework. Reprinted with permission from Burgess, D., van Ryn, M., Dovidio, J., Saha, S. (2007). Reducing racial bias among health care providers: Lessons from social cognitive psychology. *Journal of General Internal Medicine, 22*, 882–887.

emotions and can have a deleterious effect if not embedded in the understanding that holding stereotypes is natural and attempts to suppress those biases can lead to feelings and behaviors that are not conducive to best practice (e.g., resulting in practitioners being too cautious in communication or avoiding communication altogether). As has been noted elsewhere in this text, emotion plays a role in clinical practice. Whether aware of it or not, if one has implicit bias toward a particular group, that bias may be shown through what are perceived to be negative behaviors (e.g., reduced eye contact, spending less time with the client/patient). The literature in social cognitive psychology has substantiated that, for some, discomfort (as a result of implicit bias) can increase anxiety (Plant & Devine, 2003). Thus, for clinicians, this might translate into less than optimal behaviors during clinical interactions with clients/patients from an "other" group. Often, these behaviors may be nonverbal (e.g., the orientation of one's body in relation to the client/patient) and can be interpreted as dislike by the client/patient (Dovidio, Gaertner, Kawakami, & Hodson, 2002). The best strategy for addressing the discomfort or anxiety around interacting with "others" is to do just that—find and create opportunities to spend time with those who are different from yourself, socially and clinically. Increasing positive experiences with "others" will promote more positive perspectives and translate into better clinical practice. When practitioners have positive emotional responses to these experiences, they have greater capacity to be open to their clients/patients. Obviously, as human beings, we will encounter negative circumstances and people—stress in life is unavoidable. Thus, part of our growth as clinicians is to find ways in which we can regulate emotional reactions to stress. The better able we are to manage stress overall, the better the emotional state we bring to clinical work.

Additionally, Burgess et al. (2007) discuss how our orientation to "others" can be enhanced through direct work involving empathy. As self-identified "helpers," we believe we have great empathy. Although that may be true, the enrichment of empathy is something from which all of us can benefit. The literature on empathy identifies both cognitive and affective elements (Batson, 1998; Dovidio, Gaertner, Stewart, Esses, & ten Vergert, 2004): perspective taking and affective empathy. Batson (1998) has argued that perspective taking increases feelings around empathy, and those feelings, in turn, feed into the perspective taking. How does one achieve perspective taking and affective empathy? Practice, that's how. The use of imagery (i.e., imagining oneself in the "other's" situation) and role play are two strategies proposed by Burgess et al.

Practicing Empathy Exercise
After viewing this short clip on the concept of empathy: https://www.youtube.com/watch?v=1Evwgu369Jw, *identify a situation in which you felt you received sympathy from another and one in which someone responded to you with empathy. Describe how each experience made you feel.*

Finally, our orientation toward assisting those who are different from ourselves includes the building of partnerships. This process is in opposition to the traditional "expert model" of clinical practice. In the old model, the practitioner was believed to be the expert and therefore maintained a position of control and superiority. Reflecting this orientation, the clinical encounter would be driven by the practitioner and the client/patient would have a minimal role other than to respond to the direction of the practitioner. Such an interaction is not conducive to partnering and often leaves the "other" feeling even more on the outside. There is ample evidence in the psychology literature that reactions to the perception that one is "left out" or of less status lead to feelings of alienation and reduced capacity for and effectiveness in partnering together (Brewer & Brown, 1998; Fiske, 2002; Gaertner & Dovidio, 2000; Hewstone, Rubin, & Willis, 2002).

If we are truly committed to counteracting implicit bias, we will want to engage with each and every one of our clients/patients using the individuation approach. Ultimately, practices aimed at reducing implicit bias will improve our ability to provide high-quality services overall. Not only will our therapeutic approach be better tailored to the individual client/patient by following an orientation of individuation, but also our ability to develop appropriate diagnostic impressions and effective intervention paradigms and procedures will be greatly enhanced.

In Communication Sciences and Disorders

Our discipline and ASHA, through its Office of Multicultural Affairs,[3] have worked to bring multiculturalism to the forefront of education and practice. ASHA defines

---

[3] http://www.asha.org/Practice/multicultural/

cultural competence as involving "understanding and appropriately responding to the unique combination of cultural variables—including ability, age, beliefs, ethnicity, experience, gender, gender identity, linguistic background, national origin, race, religion, sexual orientation, and socioeconomic status—that the professional and client/patient bring to interactions."[4] Note that this definition reminds us that both entities (client/patient and professional) have responsibility in engaging in culturally sensitive practice. The knowledge and skills necessary for culturally sensitive practice are outlined for both audiologists and SLPs in a document written by ASHA's Multicultural Issues Board (ASHA, 2004). Among the knowledge and skills are the following:

- [Recognize the] influence of one's own beliefs and bias in providing effective services.
- Respect for an individual's race, ethnic background, lifestyle, physical/mental ability, religious beliefs/practices, and heritage.
- [Recognize the] influence of the client's/patient's traditions, customs, values, and beliefs related to providing effective services.
- [Recognize the] impact of assimilation and/or acculturation processes on the identification, assessment, treatment, and management of communication disorders/differences.
- Recognition of the clinician's own limitations in education/training in providing services to a client/patient from a particular cultural and/or linguistic community.

So, how does one gain the knowledge and skills necessary for culturally sensitive practice? And what does it look like in clinical practice? In an unpublished doctoral dissertation, Godsey (2011) explores the nature of cultural competence and professional identity development in second-year CSD graduate students. At the foundation of her research is the premise that cultural competence ". . . should not be a destination, it should be a process" (p. 3). Having said that, Godsey explores students' perspectives on cultural competence in relation to their own cultural backgrounds, the culture of the profession of speech-language pathology, their definitions of cultural competence and whether or not they consider themselves to be culturally competent. The findings indicate that these students' perspectives on cultural competence primarily involve knowledge of facts and features of certain groups and skills having to do with the application of those facts. Omitted from the orientation of the students are factors related to interactions and relationships, and although the students readily identify whether or not they are culturally competent, they are unable to provide an adequate definition of the concept of cultural competence. Further, when it comes to reflecting on clinical experiences, the students maintain a viewpoint in which "other" is defined exclusively as the client or patient. That is, they do not ". . . recognize there are differences and similarities among people

---

[4] http://www.asha.org/Practice-Portal/Professional-Issues/Cultural-Competence/

in every interaction. Instead they reference how others are different from the norm, meaning themselves" (p. 66). This highlights the remarks in the quote from Pickering (2003) in Chapter 3—that we are all a part of the diversity mix and that such a philosophy needs to be explored and reinforced throughout our education and professional lives. In response to this, Godsey recommends revising the teaching of multiculturalism and cultural competence to reflect relationship, interaction, and communication. She suggests that a shift away from learning facts about different cultures will assist student learning in three ways. First, it will help them feel less burdened by the idea that they will never know all there is to know about "other" cultures. Second, it provides the opportunity to explore multiculturalism from an integrated view, rather than an "I/we versus other" or majority versus minority approach. And, third, it allows students to see beyond what may be regional or geographic constraints. This third point is particularly salient given the ever-changing cultural make-up of our society and the continual processes of globalization.

In another study exploring cultural awareness among SLP graduate students, Howells, Barton, and Westerveld (2016) observe a relationship between academic and clinical environments with respect to learning about multiculturalism. That is, students with clinical experience are able to bring together classroom learning and practical learning in constructing a notion of cultural sensitivity. These authors use Wells' (2000) model to characterize the students' developmental stage of cultural competence and conclude they are at a point of competence because of their ability to integrate knowledge and experience in making adjustments in clinical services. Overall, the researchers stress the importance of the context (i.e., clinical setting) as essential to growth along the cultural competence continuum, and effective knowledge and skills in one context may not generalize to a different context. Therefore, students and mentors must work to facilitate the transfer of these important skills.

This brief exploration of multicultural perspectives and culturally sensitive care provides another lens through which to contemplate our approach to clinical services. The bedrock of a humanistic approach to clinical work is to regard each and every client/patient as an individual, and without examining our own perspectives, we will fall short of achieving best practice. As White (2011) asserts,

> Humanistic medicine asks the physician to organize her practice around an awareness of that patient's needs. But it also challenges the physician to undertake a further and more difficult effort—this one directed inward.

> The fundamental requirement of humanistic medicine is openness to recognizing our own biases and the desire to counteract them. Humanistic, or egalitarian medicine, asks us to candidly assess some of our most private and least acknowledged attitudes. (p. 278)

The discussion is specific to physicians and the field of medicine, however, these sentiments can be applied to any discipline of health care. More and more, both empirical and anecdotal evidence tells us that the experience of receiving health care services (including therapies) can be stressful for both patient and provider. At the same time, we know that audiologists and SLPs are among the most satisfied with their careers. We suspect the expression of satisfaction points to clinicians who work to uphold a humanistic approach to their clients and patients.

The Client/Patient

Client or patient characteristics have been identified as central to outcomes of therapeutic services (see review by Bohart & Greaves Wade, 2013). In fact, some estimate that as much as 40% of the outcome (Wampold, 2001) can be attributed to the client and factors in the client's environment (Lambert, 1992; Orlinsky, Rønnestad, & Willutzki, 2004). In their extensive review of the psychotherapy literature on client variables, Bohart and Greaves Wade (2013) point out that perspectives on how the client factors into therapy processes and outcomes have evolved from attempting to identify single factors that predict success in therapy to a more holistic point of view in which the nature of the therapeutic relationship is always changing because it is an interactive dynamic.

In considering the implications of psychotherapeutic research on client/patient factors for CSD, it is important to note at the outset that limited support exists for an effect from demographic variables, such as age or gender (e.g., Bowman, Scogin, Floyd, & McKendree-Smith, 2001; Castonguay & Beutler, 2006b; Clarkin & Levy, 2004; Cuijpers, van Straten, Smit, & Andersson, 2009). The research on cultural considerations, on the other hand, tells us these are important for the therapeutic process and outcomes, as we discussed earlier in this chapter (e.g., Castonguay & Beutler, 2006a; see also Lambert et al., 2006). Issues around severity of disorder and the presence of concomitant concerns are significant in as far as some clients will need extensive, additional, or adapted services. Thus, those involved with making decisions about resources and support available will need to keep such factors in mind. Most importantly, the research on client characteristics as predictive of outcome or instrumental in the course of treatment informs us that clients who are motivated and open to change and possess a certain capacity for mindfulness are more likely to succeed in therapy. When clients' perspectives on the therapeutic process are probed, they stress the importance of the relationship with the therapist (more on this in the following chapter on the client–clinician relationship) and how they view the nature of their psychological concerns and their investment (how hard they work, the ability to reflect, and willingness to try new things) are all seen as instrumental in their progress and success. Bohart and Greaves Ward (2013) conclude that clients often see themselves as "change agents," and their perceptions, although not always coinciding with therapist perceptions, appear to be more closely related to outcome in psychotherapy than those of the therapist. These authors suggest ". . . how they construe therapy influences what they get out of it" (p. 245).

Past research looking at client characteristics in CSD hints at a constellation of client behaviors that facilitate progress in therapy. From an interactive standpoint, clinicians have ranked behaviors, such as motivation, the client's ability to provide an appropriate response, and the level of independence in the learning process, as central to facilitating the therapeutic process (Stech, Curtiss, Troesch, & Binnie, 1973). Such characteristics are consistent with those identified in the psychotherapy literature as helpful to establishing a relationship and making progress in therapy. As stated by Oratio (1980), "While rapport has traditionally been viewed as a therapeutic atmosphere which is initially established by the clinician, the emergence of this dimension suggests that the state of rapport is clearly reflected in the clients' ongoing behavior and is regarded by supervisors as a central construct to the therapeutic process" (228). The implications of this information for clinical practice are straightforward: (1) client perspectives may differ from those of the clinician on what is happening in therapy, and therefore, (2) there is opportunity for clinicians to learn from their clients. In fact, Bohart and Greaves Ward (2013) recommend soliciting feedback each and every session, which can achieve two objectives—the collection of data/evidence and increasing the clinician's sensitivity to the evolution of treatment from the perspective of the client.

The Child as Client/Patient

In general, research investigating the features of children in treatment for speech, language, hearing, or swallowing disorders as related to treatment goals and outcomes primarily focuses on pretreatment characteristics, such as severity of impairment (e.g., Gillam et al., 2008; Petersen, Gillam, Spencer, & Gillam, 2010; Washington, Thomas-Stonell, McLeod, & Warr-Leeper, 2015). And although there is research showing that treatment works (c.f., Cirrin & Gillam, 2008; Law, Garrett, & Nye, 2004), less evidence is available attesting to specific client/patient characteristics (such as those described in the preceding paragraph) and their relationship to gains made in treatment. One such recent study of school-age children with language impairment explores the relationship between pretherapy cognitive and noncognitive measures and gains made over the course of an academic year (Justice, Jiang, Logan, & Schmitt, 2017). This study follows nearly 300 kindergarten and first-grade children identified with and receiving therapy for language impairment in public schools. The authors determine that pretherapy measures of phonological awareness, vocabulary, nonverbal cognition, and certain problem behaviors appear to be most related to gains made in language therapy. In their discussion, Justice et al. (2017) suggest that interactions between these variables may play a role in the effectiveness of treatment and/or in the ways in which clinicians conduct therapy with these youngsters. In particular, the authors point out that those children whose pretherapy scores in language (specifically phonological awareness and vocabulary) were higher tend to make greater improvements in therapy. This seems to reflect what the authors refer to as "a paradox of sorts, in that interventions serve to provide greater benefit to those who presumably need the intervention less" (p. 13). It is not the purpose of this text to review the research on intervention in language impairment, however, the results of the Justice et al. study highlight the need for a better understanding of the effects of client characteristics on treatment outcomes and how variables beyond those of communication must be considered. Experienced clinicians working with children have long known the importance of characteristics such as attention, memory, regulation, and others, as related to therapy and its outcomes. The significance of the Justice et al. findings may be in the recognition that clinicians have a duty to reflect on their practices with all children, to ensure they are providing the best possible treatment regardless of the nature of a child's speech, language, cognition, and behavior.

Another area of research involving characteristics of children receiving communication intervention is that of stuttering. Most recently, attention has focused on emotional regulation and reactivity, as well as resilience (e.g., Choi, Conture, Walden, Jones, & Kim, 2016; Caughter & Dunsmuir, 2017). These investigations suggest that children who stutter possess certain emotional predispositions that could be related to how they react to circumstances in the environment, manifesting in stuttering (Choi et al., 2016) and different responses to treatment (Caughter & Dunsmuir, 2017). Briefly, evidence is mounting that supports a model of stuttering in which emotion plays a role, whether as a result of a certain predisposition or because of momentary arousal and reaction (see Choi et al., 2016, for a review of this research). Further, Caughter and Dunsmuir (2017) identify factors that appear to be related to children who stutter making change in therapy. Among these are knowledge (understanding stuttering and speech), resilience (coming back from facing adversity), and shared experience, which came about because the children were involved in a group therapy process. Whereas knowledge and shared experience are related to the therapeutic process, other elements identified by Caughter and Dunsmuir include those present prior to therapy, such as the availability of supports, including peers.

Other examples of research on client/patient factors and therapy outcomes involve children on the autism spectrum. This work reveals connections between severity of impairment, verbal and nonverbal skills, existence of problem behaviors, and outcomes (see Steinhausen, Mohr Jensen, & Lauritsen, 2016, for a review of autism spectrum disorder [ASD] and outcomes research). Most of this research pertains to the use of measures of IQ, social skills, communication abilities, and type of intervention to "characterize" the child. Translating the research findings so that clinicians can best facilitate change suggests that children with ASD benefit best from early intervention when they exhibit some amount of basic language skills, particularly when social and adaptive behavior skills have greater impairments (e.g., Nahmias, Kase, & Mandell, 2014). Further, characteristics of anxiety, such as social fearfulness and avoidance, are related to poorer cognitive outcomes in elementary school children with ASD (Pellechia et al., 2016). Additionally, both retrospective and prospective studies of adolescents and adults with autism indicate a relationship between IQ and later outcome, although when examining those without intellectual impairment, predicting outcome is not as straightforward and may include other child-level variables, such as preponderance of repetitive behaviors, level of hyperactivity, or access to peer connections (e.g., Anderson, Liang, & Lord, 2014; Locke, Williams, Shih, & Kasari, 2017). Recent findings regarding the lack of direct correspondence between overall intellectual functioning and outcome point to the presence of adaptive functioning skills (e.g., Anderson et al., 2016), levels of anxiety and/or depression (Gillespie-Lynch et al., 2012; Tonge & Einfeld, 2003; White, Ollendick, & Bray, 2011), and differences in emotional perception (Otsuka, Uono, Yoshimura, Zhao, & Toichi, 2017) as potentially influencing overall outcome.

A review of research investigating outcomes in children with hearing loss shows considerable variability related to what is used to measure outcome, the nature of the hearing loss, and whether or not intervention involves cochlear implantation or hearing aid use. In general, studies look at the development of speech and language and/or quality of life measures to evaluate outcome in this population. Findings from these investigations identify similar factors related to outcome, such as degree and duration of hearing loss, age at hearing aid fitting or cochlear implantation along with configuration (i.e., unilateral/bilateral), maternal education, and household income (e.g., Boss, Niparko, Gaskin, & Levinson, 2011; Rachakonda et al., 2014). In a large-scale Australian study, Ching and Dillon (2013) describe outcomes at 3 years of age for 451 children diagnosed with hearing loss through newborn hearing screening and services through a national service. This group includes all children whose families agreed to participate regardless of the severity of hearing loss, presence of other impairments, or means of intervention. Factors impacting language outcome for this cohort include severity of hearing loss, the child's gender, whether or not other impairments are present, age at cochlear implantation, and the mother's level of education. In large measure, findings are consistent with what would be predicted; that is, greater hearing loss, presence of concomitant impairments, later implantation (and prescription of hearing aids), and reduced maternal education are all associated with poorer language outcomes. Of importance is the authors' interpretation relative to clinical practice urging the implementation of family-centered treatment. They state, "Parents articulated the desire for clinicians and professionals to provide them with information and ongoing support that are tailored to their individual needs" (p. S67).

To identify factors related to quality of life and hearing impairment in children living in Singapore, Looi, Lee, and Loo (2016) compare families with children using hearing aids or cochlear implants to families whose children have normal hearing. Measures of quality of life for both the children and their families show significant differences between the groups, with children with normal hearing and their families reporting better quality of life than those living with hearing loss. The authors note that parents of children with hearing aids report higher scores (meaning better quality of life) than do parents of children with cochlear implants. An examination of factors potentially related to quality of life reveals only a single significant one, that of household income. Middle-income parents reported lower quality of life scores for their children with hearing loss than did parents with high incomes. Another notable finding is that parents and their normal-hearing children present closer consistency in their ratings of quality of life as compared to pairs involving children with hearing impairment. Overall, the authors suggest that clinicians will want to make note of the impact different interventions and household income may have on perceived quality of life. The importance of this is that individual clinicians must consider these factors and modify their approach and intervention to best meet the needs of both the family and the child.

The preceding discussion of research into child characteristics and the therapeutic process contains only a few examples. The traditional approach to predicting outcome in children with communication impairments relies on drawing correlations between early measures of certain behaviors and later outcome measures. From the standpoint of identifying key child characteristics that influence the therapeutic process, such research is only so useful. As clinical observers, it is essential that we recognize influential variables, such as developmental level, presence of additional impairments, social supports, and socioeconomic factors; however, in the course of day-to-day clinical work, we will want to pay attention to components internal to the child as well. In some ways, the research on stuttering in children has begun to tease apart some of these pieces in an attempt to explain the phenomenon and development of stuttering. And, although we cannot say for certain that every child who stutters possesses a predisposition to react emotionally to communicative situations, we can remind ourselves that treatment can be adjusted to take into account more than simply speech behavior. As well, in the case of children on the autism spectrum, our work will be greatly enhanced if, as we plan and carry out therapy, we keep in mind those potentially critical factors related to a youngster's anxiety, social skill, or adaptive functioning.

The Adult as Client/Patient

Studies investigating client/patient characteristics with adults receiving speech, language, swallowing, or hearing treatment have looked at features beyond pretreatment communication status. Areas in which a fair amount of research has been conducted include aphasia, stuttering, and hearing loss. The predictive value of psychological factors on treatment outcomes is explored in a study of 50 individuals receiving outpatient speech and language therapy for chronic aphasia poststroke (Votruba, Rapport, Whitman, Johnson, & Langenecker, 2013). Of particular interest to the authors is the relationship between aspects of personality, specifically negative affectivity, as reported by both the client/patient and an individual familiar with the client/patient, and outcome of speech and language therapy. Affectivity, which can be characterized as negative or positive, reflects a person's general emotional disposition. Negative affectivity is associated with negative emotions and poor self-concept, whereas positive affectivity is reflected in calmness and confidence. Votruba et al. (2013) demonstrate a moderate relationship between affectivity and pretreatment language functioning and the gains made in therapy. Those with high negative affectivity show lower language scores and fewer gains in treatment than do individuals with high positive affectivity scores. The amount of affect that a patient expresses is also related to language skills, such that those who use affect expressively tend to have better language. The authors suggest clinicians be sure to have a full appraisal of the client's/patient's emotional and psychological functioning available to best address needs in therapy and make appropriate referrals for additional therapy (such as psychological counseling). Similar to research discussed in other sections of this text, gathering input from important people in the client's/patient's life can provide insight otherwise unavailable or not recognized by the clinician. As asserted by Votruba et al., "the caregiver is likely the best able to report on the patient's strengths and weaknesses, as well as areas of progress" (p. 428).

There is a long history of research investigating the treatment of stuttering in adults; however, a central question that often remains is determining which comes first—the stuttering followed by "characteristics" developed as a result of the stuttering (e.g., anxiety and slow response time) *or* particular "characteristics" (e.g., subtle linguistic difficulties and motor speech delays) that precipitate the stuttering. In terms of identifying characteristics central to the client's/patient's progress in treatment, agency (Plexico, Manning & Levitt, 2009) and locus of causality (Lee, Manning, & Herder, 2015) have been discussed recently. These features include the ability of a person to behave in a way different from in the past (i.e., agency) and whether or not a person is likely to choose to act rather than choose to react (i.e., locus of causality). Why discuss these concepts? Because determining the ways in which a client/patient copes with and works on a particular issue can be enormously beneficial to the therapeutic process. The literature tells us that people who stutter who express greater agency are more likely to choose action and therefore show meaningful change in treatment (Lee et al., 2015; Plexico et al., 2009). For clinical practice, measuring and being mindful of such traits in our clients help us develop therapeutic plans that match the ways in which clients work.

Research in audiology shows associations between some psychosocial factors and hearing aid outcomes (Öberg, Lunner, & Andersson, 2007). For example, Öberg et al. (2007) report that psychosocial well-being and the use of adaptive strategies for participating are associated with greater satisfaction with hearing aids. It is argued that practitioners pay attention to such factors in determining appropriate treatment. Further, research on outcomes of treatment for tinnitus shows certain patient factors appear to predict better outcomes (Kröner-Herwig, Zachriat, & Weigand, 2006; Theodoroff, Schuette, Griest, & Henry, 2014). In particular, patients who appear to have greater difficulty show larger response to intervention, and those with higher education appear to maintain progress longer than those with less education. Researchers in this field suggest that specific patient variables may not always predict the best type of treatment nor how well a patient will respond. Rather, the unique interactions between client variables, treatment type, and clinician characteristics result in varied outcomes.

Overall, the exploration of client/patient variables as related to the treatment process and outcomes reminds us that internal factors as well as external factors are important in considering best practices with our clients or patients. For children, the availability of supports in the forms of family members willing to provide stimulation and reinforcement of learning, peers providing social supports, and enriched learning environments go a long way toward facilitating the change we hope to make in therapy. In many cases, early intervention, with special attention to those who may need the greatest assistance, can foster development for any client/patient we may see. Unequivocal evidence for client/patient personality factors or psycho-social-emotional characteristics that best predict treatment outcomes is elusive and likely will remain so. That said, observing all kinds of clients and patients in the treatment process and giving ourselves the opportunity to observe change over time will help us to develop a fund of experience related to client variables that can be incorporated into our therapeutic philosophy when the time comes.

Chapter Summary

This chapter discusses factors related to both the clinician and the client and how they may impact the therapeutic process. We have explored characteristics of master clinicians—skills that develop over the course of a career through practice, continuing education, practice, interprofessional exposure, practice, expanding experiences, practice . . . you get the picture! Skilled clinicians make the time and take the effort to reflect on their practice, to improve. They are curious about their clients/patients and the world. They tailor services to the needs of individual clients/patients and include them in all aspects of the clinical process. Exquisite timing, focus, empathy, cultural sensitivity, attention to acquisition tasks, and others—these are the features of clinical work you will want to look for in your observations. How does the clinician show genuine interest in the client/patient? In setting up therapy, how does the clinician prepare for maximizing appropriate responses? How does the clinician demonstrate to family members that they are welcome and wholly part of therapy? In conducting your observations, these are the kinds of questions you will want to be asking—helping you to focus on the knowledge and skills needed to become a master clinician.

As students just starting out, we are curious about the client and see clinical observation as a way to learn more about communication disorders. Often, the observation experiences we gain as students may be our first exposure to communication impairment in "real life." We want to know. Does that person have a voice disorder? Are the behaviors I am observing consistent with ASD? What does a tympanic membrane look like when there is fluid in the middle ear? Is that what stuttering looks like? Does the child really hear the sounds? Clients/patients bring a myriad of complex backgrounds, needs, strengths, and others, to the clinical process. For us, it is important to remember that each one is unique, not a nebulous client/patient who is placing demands on us. Each one deserves an individualized treatment program. In this chapter, we reviewed examples of research reinforcing the importance of bearing in mind the individual nature of therapy. We see that psychosocial, economic, domestic, and cultural considerations are different for each client/patient and are essential to the development and delivery of an effective treatment plan.

Clinical observation is much more than learning the features of various communication disorders; rather, it is about observing the clinical process. Notice that this chapter spends less time on "the client" or "patient" than on the clinician, which is, presumably, the role that many of you are imagining yourselves taking on someday. It is the philosophy of this text to view clinical observation from a broad perspective—remember the "art and science" from Chapter 1? Observation should not be a passive activity. It is an opportunity for growth and the development of skills related to oneself as a critical thinker, problem solver, and creative being. Clinical observation can be the first step toward becoming a professional and a member of the larger education and health care worlds. The practices of speech-language pathology and audiology include so much more than understanding the various etiologies of hearing loss or signs and symptoms of genetic syndromes. As students, we spend so much time and energy amassing information—memorizing the cranial nerves and their functions, the diagnostic features of ASD, the speech characteristics of a child with cleft lip and palate, what the difference is between conductive and sensorineural hearing loss, the effects of traumatic brain injury on communication, and so on, and before we know it, we are thrown into clinic, expected to pull together a therapeutic plan, know how to use visual reinforcement audiometry, or provide an evidence-based rationale for the goals and objectives outlined for our client/patient. So much of this process happens with limited time spent considering who we are and how we are expected to engage in all of it professionally! Fortunately, for the vast majority of us, we are mentored by expert clinicians who have spent the time to reflect not only on their own clinical development (and continuing development) but also on how to best provide the supports and opportunities necessary for the next generations of clinicians. You are encouraged to consider the content and exercises in this chapter (and the entire text, for that matter) as one of those opportunities—to explore the larger picture of clinical work and how it fits with you as a reflective learner, scientific thinker, and "compassionate scientist."

Chapter Observations and Exercises

Exercise 4–1: Who Is a Master Clinician?

Consider who *your* ideal clinician might be. Identify three to five characteristics of the ideal, master clinician and jot them down. How would you define each of the characteristics? Do these describe you? If so, how might you go about expanding/strengthening/enhancing them? If not, how might you go about developing them?

Exercise 4–2: Contrasting Experienced and Inexperienced Clinicians

View the Tommy 1 and 2 videos and reflect on the differences between the graduate student clinician and the clinical supervisor. Include an entry in your Reflection Journal on the behavior(s) of the graduate student and those of the clinician—thinking about some of the characteristics we've discussed in this chapter and remembering to use one of the models we've discussed in earlier chapters and exercises. What impact do these behaviors have on the client? On the progress of the session? What might you take away from these observations for your own growth as an aspiring clinician?

Exercise 4–3: Expanding Our Cultural Sensitivity

Project Implicit is an organization and collaboration among researchers interested in learning about our social cognition as it functions implicitly (not at the level of conscious awareness).[5] Through their work, several assessments of "hidden" implicit bias have been developed. Log on to the website and select at least two assessments to complete. Record in your Reflection Journal what assessments you completed, how you scored, and your reaction to the experience.

Exercise 4–4: Observing Client/Patient Characteristics

In your next observation, identify three to four characteristics of the client/patient you are observing. For each characteristic, include at least two pieces of evidence that support your observation. Remember to keep in mind the difference between objective and subjective descriptions.

Exercise 4–5: A Personal Experience

Remember and describe an experience of being in a physical, social, architectural, psychological, intellectual, or cultural space that made you feel excluded. This space was not designed for you or you were not welcome in it.[6]

---

[5] https://implicit.harvard.edu/implicit/aboutus.html
[6] Adapted from Peterkin (2016).

The Client–Clinician Relationship (The Therapeutic Alliance)

Chapter Outline

I. Therapeutic Alliance in Mental Health
II. Therapeutic Alliance in Allied Health
III. Therapeutic Alliance in Communication Sciences and Disorders
    A. Therapeutic Alliance in Audiology
    B. Therapeutic Alliance in Speech-Language Pathology
IV. A Note About the ICF and the Therapeutic Alliance
    A. Clinically Significant Change
V. Chapter Summary
VI. Chapter Observations and Exercises

Learning Objectives

- The reader will identify key components of the therapeutic alliance.
- The reader will describe the three elements of the International Classification of Functioning, Disability, and Health (ICF): impairment, disability, handicap.
- The reader will identify factors related to clinically significant change.
- The reader will describe ways of coping related to making change.

I propose that the working alliance between the person who seeks change and the one who offers to be a change agent is one of the keys, if not the key, to the change process.
—Bordin (1979, p. 252)

Returning to our "Ways of Knowing" framework, we see both scientific and humanistic practices. In the progression of medical care, it has only been in the recent past (since the 19th century) that scientific health care, with its focus on disease and curing, has been dominant. Until that time, medicine was concerned with illness, caring, and healing. Some see what amounts to a pendulum swinging from one extreme (complete humanistic focus, no scientific evidence) to the other (complete scientific focus, no consideration of individual patient). And some see a health care system that is desperately in need of greater balance (e.g., Halstead, 2001). Halstead (2001) reasons that rehabilitation medicine and its allied health disciplines are, perhaps, ahead of the curve on realizing this equilibrium:

> Although professionals in any specialty can practice a blend of humanistic and scientific medicine, rehabilitation as a field is uniquely suited to achieving this balance. From its inception, the philosophy of rehabilitation has been strongly oriented toward the humanistic approach while developing an ever-expanding scientific and research base. (p. 150)

In many ways, it is up to the practitioner to make this happen, with the therapeutic alliance encompassing the client-/patient-centered approach. "There is a growing body of evidence that the quality of the therapeutic alliance is linked to the success of treatment across a broad section of clients, treatments, and identified problems" (Flückiger, Del Re, Wampold, Symonds, & Horvath, 2012, p. 10). Although this quote comes from the mental health literature, it can be applied to most relationships between health care and rehabilitation providers and their clients/patients. For example, the phrase "working alliance" has been applied to the nature of career counseling relationships (Whiston, Rossier, & Hernandez Barón, 2016). Bordin (1979) proposes that the working alliance includes three essential elements: (1) agreed-upon goals, (2) assigned tasks, and (3) an established bond between the provider and the client. In articulating the nature of these components, Bordin points out that different therapists will have different emphases in terms of the expectations of agreed-upon goals. According to Whiston et al. (2016), goals represent the degree to which agreement exists between the client and counselor on what needs to be addressed. Tasks refer to the activities that the clinician and client understand to be best in advancing the process toward the agreed-upon goals. The bond, or relationship, between the client and clinician is what makes the work necessary for achievement of the goals possible.

Therapeutic Alliance in Mental Health

Those who have studied outcomes in mental health and psychotherapy note one of the principal features predicting outcome is the therapeutic alliance (Horvath,

Del Re, Flückiger, & Symonds, 2011). Ulvenes et al. (2012) assert that, although different theoretical orientations have different stances on the value of the alliance and the role of each component (i.e., goals, tasks, bond), there is agreement that it is the alliance itself that is key to success in treatment, and importantly, ". . . the therapist is critical to making the alliance therapeutic . . ." (p. 292). An investigation of therapist ability in alliance formation with clients from counseling and psychological services in institutions of higher education reveals that the therapist is vital to the therapeutic alliance; however, variability in therapists' abilities to establish this bond appears to mediate therapeutic outcomes more so than do client variables (Baldwin, Wampold, & Imel, 2007; Del Re, Flückiger, Horvath, Symonds, & Wampold, 2012). Namely, the outcomes of therapeutic processes with therapists who have difficulty establishing or maintaining the alliance are less positive than those in which a stronger therapeutic alliance is present.

Further research into the therapeutic alliance and treatment outcomes suggests a complex relationship among the various components of the alliance (Ulvenes et al., 2012). A systematic review of research involving client–/patient–provider alliance and communication effects on adherence with mental health treatment determines that those with stronger alliance and communication between therapist and client have better adherence (Thompson & McCabe, 2015). The best approach to communication observed in the literature appears to be a collaborative one in which goals and tasks are determined and decided together by the client and the clinician. Further, a practitioner who pays close attention to questions may also facilitate greater engagement on the part of the client/patient. Elements of the alliance impact each other such that actions on the part of the therapist effect the bond, and the bond effects how the goals and tasks are determined, which subsequently impacts client behavior, therapist action, and the evolving relationship.

Therapeutic Alliance in Allied Health

Client or patient centeredness is fundamental to framing the therapeutic alliance. Tickle-Degnen (2002) discusses client-centered practice in occupational therapy as related to the therapeutic alliance by identifying two types of relationships involved—rapport and the working alliance. Rapport, as described by Rogers (1957), includes the development of a positive relationship in which the client and the clinician like each other and have feelings of respect and warmth toward each other. The working alliance, as we have previously defined, incorporates goal setting, task identification, and the bond between the client and the clinician.

Tickle-Degnen and Gavett (2003), an occupational therapist and a speech-language pathologist (SLP), propose that the foundation of a healthy and productive therapeutic alliance must include the use of specific communication strategies that vary over the course of a developing alliance. They discuss the development of the therapeutic relationship as having an initial period in which rapport is established, a second period in which the working alliance is established, and a third period, which involves maintenance of the working relationship until the goals of therapy are attained. Initially, as rapport is being established, communication strategies are used for collecting information, indicating "cooperative intent," and "regulating involvement." These strategies are used by both the client/patient and the clinician and both are equal participants in the therapeutic alliance.

In the process of developing rapport, it is the clinician's responsibility to collect information regarding the client/patient's concerns, needs, and values (in other words, the individual's perspective), along with communicating information about her or his approach to treatment, including an appropriate level of evidence regarding therapy. "Cooperative intent" refers to the expression of interest and commitment to working with the client/patient, along with recognizing the client's/patient's expectation to work together. Importantly, Tickle-Degnen (2002) states that it is vital for all involved in the working alliance to come to an agreed-upon understanding. The development of this understanding begins with the clinician communicating with the client/patient in a respectful manner, fully recognizing the client's/patient's preferences, knowledge, and skills (Tickle-Degnen, 2002). The third strategy, used early in the process of establishing rapport, is that of regulating involvement. In essence, this reflects back to one of Goldberg's (1997) master clinician skills, that of *exquisite timing*. In recognizing the client's or patient's knowledge and capabilities (as well as preferences), the expert clinician knows when or if the individual is ready for specific or more information and how to present it. Moving therapy along relative to expectations of the client's willingness and capabilities requires an understanding of how to regulate involvement. The client/patient regulates involvement through the manner in which she or he responds, including the use of direct questions, comments, and actions.

The second phase in the progression of a working alliance focuses on therapy tasks, including selection of goals and learning activities, progress, and setbacks. Through this work and continuing evolution of rapport, a culture of working together emerges (Tickle-Degnen, 2002, refers to this as a "working relational culture"). The working relational culture is the result of many interactions between the client/patient and therapist while they come to agree on goals, tasks, means of reinforcement, priorities, and a mutual understanding of the three components of evidence-based practice—client preferences, clinician expertise, and scientific evidence.

The third phase, "ongoing working relationship," is marked by the use of explicit communication. Most likely, at this point in the relationship, the therapeutic bond is strong enough that fluctuations in behavior, thoughts, and emotions will have occurred. Tickle-Degnen suggests this time in the therapeutic process requires management of these fluctuations, which can be done successfully through communication (Tickle-Degnen & Gavett, 2003). In particular, attention to emotional and interpersonal influences and the use of adaptation are important to sustaining the alliance. Throughout the therapeutic process, the client and clinician share information that allows for progression and it is important this practice continue. Again, the driving maxim should be the alliance, a partnership that allows for constant check-ins and modifications as necessary.

Emotions and thoughts about the impairment, therapy, and the future may well be expressed from the beginning of the therapeutic relationship, but often, it is not until a sense of stability in the therapeutic bond is achieved that clients/ patients feel free to communicate them. A master clinician provides the context in which emotions and thoughts can be expressed without evaluation (Luterman, 2017) and uses techniques to help manage these. For example, humor has been studied in therapy with adults with aphasia (Simmons-Mackie & Schultz, 2003). In this instance, the use of humor by both the client and the clinician is examined during the course of intervention for aphasia. The authors note that the vast majority of humor is initiated by the clinician, although there is a mutual sharing of humorous experiences and clients use more nonverbal humor than do the clinicians. When analyzed for theme, humor appears to be used for three essential purposes: to help build a bond between the client and clinician, to minimize embarrassment or make light of a potentially difficult situation, and to facilitate cooperation in therapeutic endeavors. In drawing conclusions about their findings, Simmons-Mackie and Schultz (2003) suggest that humor can be a valid component in therapy and play an important role in relationship building. Second, the authors encourage clinicians to push their clients to use humor more often, as it may be an avenue through which clients/patients gain communicative confidence and greater social skill. Further suggestions include fostering the use of nonverbal humor and reinforcing the positive impact humor can have on overall feelings. The overall message from the research can be summed in the following comment, ". . . therapists should feel comfortable having fun during the serious business of communication therapy" (Simmons-Mackie & Schultz, 2003, p. 763).

And, finally, all therapeutic processes necessitate adaptation. At the very core of therapy is change, and the process of change frequently requires adaptation. Although the focus of change in treatment may be the client/patient, there is considerable likelihood that the clinician, also, will end up changing as a result of the therapeutic alliance. Facilitating adaptation in therapy means revisiting goals, activities, progress, priorities, etc. In doing this, the clinician depends on client/ patient perspective as much as the client/patient relies on the clinician. In many ways, it is this reciprocity and mutual trust that define the alliance.

Additional work in occupational therapy and physical therapy demonstrates the significance of the working relationship. Palmadottir (2006) points out that, in a typical biophysical model (otherwise known as the medical model or expert model), the relationship between the practitioner and the patient/client is not equal. That is because the therapist, who can be seen as having all of the knowledge and expertise, is the one to determine the nature of the work to be done—to the patient/client. Research in related allied health fields shows that therapeutic relationships that are based on mutual support and uplift the client/patient are much more likely to engender positive rehabilitation experiences than are relationships that do not support the partnership (Palmadottir, 2006). Client perspectives highlight the differences between their relationships with rehabilitation specialists (e.g., occupational therapists and physical therapists) and other health professionals, in large measure because of the nature of the relationships—they tend to be less formal, are more frequent, and are individualized (Palmadottir, 2006). In interviews with 20 patients who had received occupational therapy, Palmadottir (2006) asked about the nature of their treatment and their relationship with the therapist. Identified are seven "dimensions" of the relationship, which Palmadottir describes in positive terms: concern, direction, fellowship, guidance, and coalition; a negative term: rejection; and a neutral term: detachment. Briefly, the positive dimensions are interpreted as reflecting a "trusting connection, rapport, communication, empathy and respect" and a feeling of collaboration (Palmadottir, 2006, p. 399). In elaborating on the implications of these dimensions, Palmadottir suggests that, whereas collaboration (i.e., fellowship, guidance, and coalition) is consistent with a partnership between the client/patient and therapist, the dimensions of concern and direction are associated with more control on the part of the therapist. For some interviewees, this model appears to provide comfort and a feeling of safety.

Research tells us that not all clients/patients will engage in the therapeutic process equally, and for many, they may not have much of an expectation to participate at the level of decision-making (Lund, Tamm, & Bränholm, 2001; Pellat, 2004). Still, the alliance can be successful and mutually satisfying. With respect to the other dimensions, Palmadottir (2006) notes that detachment and rejection are infrequent behaviors, but the observation of them is associated with client feelings of reduced self-esteem and fear. More importantly, the balance of the relationship and partnership can mean the difference between clients/patients not progressing, dropping out, or moving out of therapy and on with their lives with more or less autonomy and self-efficacy for decision making on their own (Pellat, 2004).

A more recent study of patient–professional relationships in occupational therapy identifies five elements that may contribute to the success of a working alliance (Morrison & Smith, 2013). Morrison and Smith (2013) find that interpersonal connection, humor as therapeutic strategy, an impetus to act leading to functional gains, a shared sense of success and patient self-efficacy (belief in one's ability to succeed), and goal achievement all advance the therapeutic alliance. These authors argue that deliberate concentration on each component of the alliance—goals, tasks, and therapeutic bond—will serve to enhance the experience for both clinician and client/patient. Therapists would do well to work on the interpersonal nature of the process, facilitative communication, and reflection skills and consider the inclusion of humor in the therapy process.

Therapeutic Alliance in Communication Sciences and Disorders

Early investigation of the relationship between the clinician and client/patient in CSD looks at the characteristics of the interactants (e.g., Haynes & Oratio, 1978; Oratio, 1980; Oratio & Hood, 1977). Valuable information from these investigations is what Oratio (1980) observes as a possible trend from paying close attention to certain technical aspects of the therapy process toward more interpersonal aspects. More recent studies of the therapeutic relationship in CSD identify specific features that appear to facilitate the process of change for many clients and patients. This literature is reviewed first in the area of audiology and then speech-language pathology.

Therapeutic Alliance in Audiology

Erdman (2013) states,

> To say that audiologists manage hearing impairment or that we manage patients with hearing impairment, in reality misses the mark. The audiologist's responsibility is to establish a therapeutic relationship and facilitate adjustment to hearing impairment by engaging patients in the actual management of their hearing problems. (p. 159)

In promoting a working alliance with clients/patients in audiologic rehabilitation, Erdman (2013) makes the case for using the biopsychosocial approach. In particular, she argues for the use of counseling as the context within which all activities relative to working with clients/patients with hearing loss are conducted. That being said, the breadth of the application of patient-centered care in audiology is not well known (e.g., Grenness, Hickson, Laplante-Levesque, & Davidson, 2014). In applying the biopsychosocial model to audiology practice, Erdman incorporates the use of narrative and empathy to facilitate the therapeutic relationship. She presents a model that includes three phases of advancement in the working alliance (see Figure 5–1). These phases represent considerable integration of research from disciplines, such as mental health counseling. Similar to that presented by Tickle-Degnen and Gavett (2003), in the first phase, the clinician and patient/client establish rapport. This is facilitated by empathic behavior on the part of the clinician, largely within the context of the patient/client telling her or his story (the narrative). As well, the clinician provides information to the patient/client to assist in her or his understanding of hearing loss and its implications and treatment. Erdman describes this as the "audiologist's cognitive and affective communications," and these are represented on the figure by the solid arrows pointing toward the "Phase 1" level.

The inclusion of the "patient's story" (or narrative) reflects Engel's (1977) "inner viewing" or reflection, but of the patient/client, rather than the clinician. He states, ". . . listening to the stories our patients share with us is precisely how we become acquainted with our patient's inner lives . . . Clinical inquiry, after all, involves nothing less than the study of one person by another, intrinsically a collaborative enterprise" (Engel, 1996, p. 434). The use of narrative, or patient/client stories, is recognized as an integral, cost-effective, and essential component of quality health care, leading to greater patient satisfaction (Charlton, Dearing, Berry, & Johnson, 2008; Epstein et al., 2003) and reduced need for diagnostic processes (Margalit & El-Ad, 2008; Margalit, Glick, Benbassat, & Cohen, 2004; Soler & Okkes, 2012). In fact, an entire field of study has emerged around "narrative health

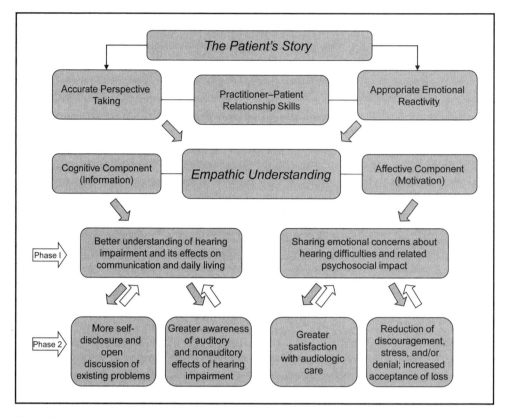

Figure 5–1. Phases in the development of the therapeutic alliance in audiologic rehabilitation. Reprinted with permission from Erdman, S. A. (2013). The biopsychosocial approach in patient- and relationship-centered care: Implications for audiologic counseling. In J. Montano & J. Spitzer (Eds.), *Adult audiologic rehabilitation* (2nd ed., pp. 159–206). San Diego, CA: Plural Publishing.

care" (Brown, Thornton, & Stewart, 2012; Charon, 2006; Engel, Zarconi, Pethtel, & Missimi, 2008; Meza & Passermann, 2011). In a brief study of undergraduate students, Berg, Canellas, Salbod, and Velayo (2008) determine that students exposed to narratives of disability and hearing loss show greater capacity for empathy and incorporate more emotion, along with technical aspects, into their understanding of the implications of hearing loss. Further, the authors suggest that exposure to narratives assists in the development of active listening skills in audiology undergraduates. This research reminds us that the practitioner's skills with communication and interpersonal connections are essential to establishing and maintaining the working alliance so critical to positive outcomes. Erdman (2013) points out that practitioners who make use of narrative are providing the opportunity to ". . . (a) elicit the patient's perspective, (b) provide an empathic response, and (c) engage the patient in the decision-making process" (p. 166).

In the second phase of Erdman's approach, the working alliance has been established, allowing the interactive nature of the relationship. In Figure 5–1, arrows representing the client/patient (open arrows) allow more disclosure regarding the nature and impact of the hearing problem, whereas the solid arrows (the audiologist) use these disclosures to provide information that fits the needs of the client/patient and they begin to form a shared understanding of the problem. On the affective side, the open arrows (client/patient) represent responses to the clinician's empathy, leading to greater satisfaction with services and a process of acceptance for the client/patient.

Phase 3 shows progress on the part of the client/patient in accepting the hearing problem and understanding its impact, communicatively and psychosocially. According to the model, this level of understanding and acceptance is related to greater consistency with treatment follow-through, which ultimately provides greater overall client/patient satisfaction and increased effectiveness of the treatment. In audiology, evidence exists for differences in how clients and clinicians view the process of hearing aid purchase decisions. For clinicians, a client's readiness for hearing aid adoption is seen as important, whereas for clients, having the clinician understand and meet the client's needs, showing support for the client's choices, and providing information are more important (Poost-Foroosh, Jennings, & Cheesman, 2015). The authors interpret the findings as indicative of the client's desire to be involved with the clinician in decision making.

There are few other studies of audiological services and the therapeutic relationship. Evaluation of communication between audiologists and clients/patients being seen for consultation, assessment, and management shows reduced patient-centered communication among audiologists (Grenness, Hickson, Laplante-Lévesque, Meyer, & Davidson, 2015a, 2015b). In particular, the authors note that communication during history-taking typically covers appropriate technical content including medical and lifestyle information; however, the communication exchange is clinician driven and involves little emotional content. Concern is expressed as to how the nature of the communication might impact later aspects of the consultation, such as treatment or management (Grenness et al., 2015a). These same investigators examine the communication patterns of 26 audiologists in 62 instances of audiologic rehabilitation consultation (Grenness et al., 2015b). Results show that, again, the nature of the interaction is clinician centered, marked by the majority of talking being done by the audiologist, focusing on treatment. In most cases, the client/patient is minimally involved in management decisions, as the majority of clinicians recommend hearing aids with little input from the client. The authors find that if more time is taken during diagnosis and planning, more patient/client involvement is observed. It is suggested that opportunities for including the clients and their companions do present themselves, but audiologists are unlikely to take advantage of them. While the research is still to be conducted, it is speculated that the lack of patient centeredness likely impacts the success of the outcome in these encounters (Grenness et al., 2015b). Interestingly, a subgroup of these investigators reports relatively high patient centeredness (as measured by a standardized instrument) among audiologists in Australia and likens their scores on subscales of *sharing* and *caring* to those of "medical practitioners" as assessed in other studies. They also note that increased age and length

of experience, along with practice settings that are related to teaching, community education, and industrial audiology appear to be related to higher scores of
patient centeredness (Laplante-Lévesque, Hickson, & Grenness, 2014).

The concept of client–/patient–clinician partnering in audiology is reiterated
in the few publications available. For example, Laplante-Lévesque, Hickson, and
Worrall (2010) report that trust in both the individual and the profession by
the client/patient is central to shared decision making. Cobelli, Gill, Cassia, and
Ugolini (2014) stress the importance of recognizing social or societal pressures
regarding hearing aid adoption as instrumental in decision making. They suggest
that practitioners take a "consumer-centric" approach, focusing on providing information and support as to the use of hearing aids, rather than solely focusing
on the product. Further, Cobelli et al. propose audiologists integrate educating
and supporting clients/patients with addressing attitudes about hearing aids so as
to reduce negative societal influences.

To conclude this section on the therapeutic relationship in audiology practice,
discussion of an additional study is warranted. To this point, we have examined
the therapeutic relationship in audiologic rehabilitation in the adult population. A
recent study of families with children who had received cochlear implants reveals
important information regarding relationship building with all family members
(Roberts, Sands, Gannoni, & Marciano, 2015). Thematic analyses of interviews
conducted with parents of cochlear implant recipients reveal three significant
themes relating to parents' concerns and needs. The first theme is that of a new
world in which the family had now entered. The notion of unfamiliarity is important, as we know this can often evoke feelings of fear. And fear can be manifested
in ways that may or may not facilitate growth in the "new world." Some parents
liken it to a "journey"—identifying the lasting nature of the change in their families' lives. The second theme relates to how services meet or do not meet the
needs of the family, particularly those of the parents. In the interviews, parents
report greater need for technical support, as well as better information tailored
to their needs, and advanced professional services. Finally, parents express value
in the development of additional connections and relationships with others in
similar circumstances. The authors recommend that audiologists work to address
the needs not only of the children receiving the implants but also those of their
parents.

Overall, the working alliance or therapeutic relationship in audiology reflects
that of other allied health disciplines. A biopsychosocial approach helps to put the
research into context and provide a framework with which the audiologist can
practice. In summarizing the biopsychosocial approach to audiologic services,
Erdman (2013) states:

> The biopsychosocial approach, as manifested in patient- and relationship-
> centered care, places counseling at the forefront of intervention as the founda-
> tion of audiology's therapeutic context, therapeutic process, and therapeutic
> activities. . . . By establishing an empathic, facilitative relationship with pa-
> tients, audiologists will be able to promote patients' self-advocacy and engage

them in a mutual decision making process regarding the optimal management of their hearing problems. The outcome of successful audiologic care will be patients who are able to manage their hearing-related communication and psychosocial problems effectively and who are satisfied with the audiologic care we have provided. (pp. 195–196)

Therapeutic Alliance in Speech-Language Pathology

Using the key words and phrases of *therapeutic alliance* or *therapeutic relationship* and *speech-language pathology* in an online search of MEDLINE, PsychInfo, and CINAHL reveals very few resources. What has been written about the therapeutic alliance appears, primarily, in literature related to aphasia therapy, stuttering, and/or the ending of the therapeutic process (i.e., dismissal from therapy or death). One of the earliest references to the therapeutic alliance in speech-language pathology appears in a brief article by Hooper (1996) in which she discusses the use of an "ecomap" in conducting treatment with older adults with aphasia. The ecomap is a tool, often used by social workers, to identify the important support people in a client's life, such as spouse, children, neighbors, friends, and others. Hooper suggests drawing out a map in which the closeness of the relationship and the communication connections can be illustrated, thereby assisting the client/patient with memory, recognizing valuable relationships, and communication. Either with the client/patient directly or with family and others who are significant to the client, the clinician can help determine how each person interacts and communicates with family members and the impact on the quality of life of the client/patient. In this fashion, Hooper makes a pitch for including those important relationships as therapeutic and, thus, part of the alliance. Harkening back to our discussion of cultural sensitivity and competence, Hooper's discussion reminds the practitioner that perspectives on age and illness carry their own biases and cultures, and it is important that we assess our own stereotypes and be mindful of them when working with older adults. An example of an ecomap for "Rick," who is 64 years old and experiencing aphasia following a stroke, is presented in Figure 5–2. The map contains circles representing the significant relationships in his life where communication is important to him. The thickness of the arrows represents the strength of the relationship and the density of the pattern in each arrow represents the difficulty of the communication. Thus, we see that both Rick and his wife Cheryl express great strength in their relationship, but their impressions of the ease with which they communicate differ. Rick finds it more difficult to communicate with Cheryl than she does in communicating with Rick. The ecomap also shows us that Cheryl has very strong ties with her parents and her book club. Rick expresses stronger communicative connections with friends and family around recreation. Overall, there appear to be fewer stronger relationships and more difficult communicative connections for Rick than for Cheryl, which is not surprising. The benefit of using the ecomap is that it allows all involved to identify the key relationships and communicative situations that are of greatest

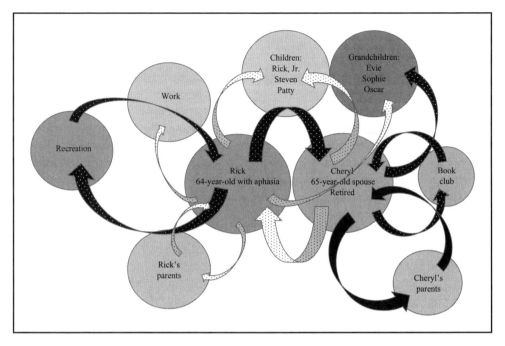

Figure 5–2. Example ecomap.

importance. Having this visual image provides a starting place for determining priorities in therapy.

Early research on the therapeutic relationship in speech-language pathology focuses on skill development and clinical experience and their connection to counseling behavior (F'arkington & Rae, 1996), as well as factors identified by speech-language pathologists as important to therapeutic outcomes (Adamson, Hand, Heard, & Nordholm, 1999). Both of these studies use methods involving the surveying of SLPs. F'arkington and Rae (1996) determine that counseling, as a concept, is understood by both SLP students and experienced clinicians, whereas behaviors associated with counseling are more likely to be observed in experienced clinicians and less so in students. The authors contend there is value in the pursuit of personal therapy on the part of practitioners, which can contribute to the making of a healthy therapeutic relationship between clients/patients and SLPs. In their survey of Australian SLPs examining factors that facilitate therapeutic outcomes, Adamson et al. (1999) show that SLPs identify a "positive therapeutic relationship" as key to better outcomes. This finding, along with other related factors noted in the study, is interpreted as indicative of a humanistic approach to the therapeutic process.

More recently, explorations of the therapeutic relationship among patients/clients with aphasia or acquired communication and swallowing disorders have focused on the perspectives of those with the impairment or their caregivers (Burns, Baylor, Dudgeon, Starks, & Yorkston, 2015; Fourie, 2009; McClellan,

McCann, Worrall, & Harwood, 2014). People with neurologic communication disorders are at considerable disadvantage when accessing and making use of therapeutic services (e.g., Burns et al., 2015). Coming to appreciate the limitations and barriers experienced by the patient/client is essential for a humanistic approach to therapy. Fourie (2009) presents the perspectives of people with acquired communication and swallowing disorders after having interviewed them as to their responses to a set of four questions. The questions addressed the patients' experiences with speech, language, and swallowing therapy; whether or not their expectations were met; which aspects of the clinician's approach were particularly helpful; and what advice they might have for future clinicians. Further, he solicits narratives from the patients as to their best and worse therapy sessions. From these interviews, Fourie organizes the comments into categories of "therapeutic actions" and "therapeutic qualities," revealing four actions and four qualities. The therapeutic actions are described as "confident," "soothing," "practical," and "empowering," whereas therapeutic qualities include "understanding," "graciousness," "erudition," and "inspiration." The qualities identified by the clients/patients are seen as providing support and the actions of the clinicians identified are cognitive or emotive behaviors seen as supporting. The power of this study is that it directly reflects client or patient perspectives, and it may have direct clinical applicability. Fourie summarizes by suggesting students of SLP learn about the contributions clinicians make to the therapeutic relationship—focusing on ". . . *how* therapy is conducted rather than . . . on *what* therapy is conducted" (italics in original, pp. 996–997).

In a related study, Burns et al. (2015) interviewed people with neurologic communication disorders and one of their family members, as well as physicians who treated adult patients. In particular, the researchers' interests lie in how patients and families perceive communication with the medical community as compared to how physicians perceive communication with patients with communication impairment. Analysis of the interview data reveal three themes, two related to the patients and family members and one related to the physicians. As can be seen in Table 5–1, patients and their families consider themselves a "team" and they expect doctors to at least try to communicate with them. Physicians, in turn, want to communicate with their patients but feel they do not know how. Key subthemes that emerge from these data are that patients want to try their hand at communicating but also recognize that having a family member present helps. As for their expectations of physicians, both patients and family members express disappointment and frustration with communication at times and question whether or not some physicians even want to make the effort to communicate. One of the unique contributions of this research is that of the family member perspective. In large measure, family members perceive themselves as part of a team, rather than an uninvolved resource, such as an interpreter. They appear to take on a number of roles relative to communication, and these roles change as the patient's communication capabilities change. Most family members report taking on responsibilities that assist both the patient and the physician. Examples are modeling for the physician how to speak with the patient, providing content

Table 5–1. Themes and Subthemes Expressed by Individuals With Aphasia, Family Members, and Physicians

Theme	Subtheme
1. Patients and family members are a team.	1–1. The team works together.
	1–2. Patients "want to try."
	1–3. Family members help it "go smoother."
	1–4. Teams can change.
	1–5. Teams can sometimes struggle.
2. Patients and family members want physicians to "just try."	2–1. Communicating with physicians is hard.
	2–2. We feel some physicians may not know or may not try.
	2–3. Poor communication can damage the relationship between the team and the physician.
	2–4. How communication should be.
3. Physicians want to try but may not know how.	3–1. Effective communication is our responsibility.
	3–2. Communication with patients is hard.
	3–3. We rely on family members.
	3–4. We are not taught how to do it.

Source: Reprinted with permission from Burns, Baylor, Dudgeon, Starks, and Yorkston (2015). Asking the stakeholders: Perspectives of individuals with aphasia, their family members, and physicians regarding communication in medical interactions. *American Journal of Speech-Language Pathology*, 24, 341–357.

to the physician for the patient who is unable to or has become fatigued, and advocating for the patient. Although therapy for a population such as the one discussed in the Burns et al. study has moved toward making the environment more "communicatively accessible," the authors suggest tailoring treatment to include strategies aimed at specific communicative interactions, such as medical consultations. They point out that SLPs should be providing direct communication training to those who are assisting patients, whether they be family members, medical advocates, or physicians.

Additional research on the therapeutic alliance in SLP has been conducted in the area of adult stuttering therapy (Gerlach & Subramanian, 2016; Manning, 2010; Plexico, Manning, & DiLollo, 2010). Gerlach and Subramanian (2016) investigated the effects of "bibliotherapy" on the therapeutic process in adults who stutter working with graduate clinicians. The authors define bibliotherapy as ". . . the process of reading, reflecting upon, and discussing literature, often first person illness or disability narratives, to promote cognitive shifts in the way clients and clinicians conceptualize the experience of disability" (p. 2). Much like narrative training in medical student education, the process of using literature in therapy can be facilitative of growth not only in clients/patients, but also in CSD students. In the Gerlach and Subramanian study, the clinicians, none of whom stuttered, express increased rapport and a stronger therapeutic alliance as a result of the bibliotherapy experience.

Through an exhaustive, qualitative approach to determining the therapeutic experience of adults who stutter, Plexico et al. (2010) identify the characteristics cited by clients as most related to effectiveness in stuttering therapy. In doing so, they note key components of the therapeutic process, along with specific qualities of effective clinicians. These aspects, together, are described as elements of a successful therapeutic alliance. The authors state, "At the core . . . was the clinician's skill in demonstrating to the client a passion for assisting them . . . communicating their understanding of the . . . experience of stuttering . . . the willingness . . . to listen carefully . . . and to focus on the client's unique goals and capabilities" (p. 348). Engaging with this type of clinician results in greater "motivation, acceptance, understanding and trust" on the part of the client. Further, the authors caution that clients who related a negative therapeutic experience (i.e., limited change) viewed their clinicians as lacking competence because they were unable to provide adequate rationale for their therapeutic choices; did not consider the clients' needs, desires, or input; and frequently communicated judgment, lack of interest, and impatience. The resulting feelings engendered in the clients by ineffective clinicians include a whole host: frustration, shame, hopelessness, inadequacy, embarrassment, anger, and discouragement (Plexico et al., 2010). Although these findings reflect the experiences and opinions of clients who stutter, they are applicable to all therapeutic interactions. Moreover, Plexico et al. recommend the use of client/patient feedback as central to maintaining a positive therapeutic alliance. The conclusions put forth by these authors should be considered a "wake-up" call to all practitioners that clinical expertise matters. Recall, the effective clinician makes use of reflection to continually improve her or his therapeutic practice. In the case of both reflection and specific clinical knowledge and skills, advancement is incumbent on the clinician—to become a master clinician, who is considered successful at establishing an effective therapeutic alliance and fostering change, one must be willing to engage in continual self and professional growth.

We now move to looking at the therapeutic alliance in speech-language pathology as evidenced in treatment with children. Again, few studies examine the experiences of children in speech and language therapy and their families relative to the therapeutic alliance (e.g., Fourie, Crowley, & Oliviera, 2011). Drawing from the mental health literature, researchers have hinted at connections between a child's mental well-being and her or his ability to communicate (e.g., Danger & Landreth, 2005). Certainly, this has implications for the therapeutic alliance in speech and language therapy in children. Past research indicates that many children are aware of communication impairment, either in themselves or in others, and they also recognize the impact such difficulties can have on relationships with peers (see Shirk & Karver, 2003). Thinking about the nature of communication impairment and its potential impact on young children, I recall something a colleague of mine said in reference to the children with whom she was working. This SLP worked in a "total communication" program in which children who were deaf and other hearing children with developmental language disorder were together in a preschool class in which all communication was done both orally and using American Sign Language. She noted that, even at 3 and 4 years of age, these groups of children demonstrated different social behaviors. The children with deafness often expressed themselves in animated ways, by any means they could, to both peers and adults. In contrast, the SLP described many of the children with language impairment as considerably more subdued and reticent to communicate. In contemplating the reasons for these differences, we speculated that, in part, the children with hearing impairment or deafness had some understanding as to why they did not communicate in the same way as other children, whereas the children with language impairment experienced a frustration coming from an awareness of the difficulties but a lack of clear explanation regarding why they experienced communication challenges. Thus, as clinicians working with these children, the vast majority for whom we will not know why communication is impaired, much of our job may involve helping these youngsters feel safe enough to try to communicate.

Fourie et al. (2011) provide one of the only recent studies directly examining children's perspectives on the therapeutic relationship in speech-language pathology. By interviewing six children (ages 5–12 years) in speech-language therapy, Fourie et al. sought to conceptualize the "life-worlds" of these children's therapeutic experiences. The concept of a life-world comes from Husserl (1970) and concerns the ". . . often taken-for-granted, subjective experiences that help constitute human social reality" (Fourie et al., 2011, p. 314). Thematic analyses of the children's responses reveal six topics relating to the therapeutic relationship: play/fun, differences in power, trust, routines/rituals, role confusion, and physical features of the clinician. Play is the realm through which young children do their learning, and it is mentioned by children in therapy as essential to a quality experience. The authors point out that not only does play facilitate learning and self-regulation in children, but it also can be vital to the establishment of a bond between therapist and child. Thus, its importance cannot be understated. Differences in power is another theme to have emerged. A working relationship in which the clinician has all of the power can result in reduced engagement in the process on the part of the client (Ferguson & Armstrong, 2004). Trust carries a great deal of weight in the therapeutic alliance, whether the client/patient is a child or adult. For children, clinicians who provide options and choices, while maintaining routine, safety, and trust, are much more likely to have strong bonds with their clients. In cases in which the child loses trust in the clinician, the bond may suffer. Fourie et al. share a story about "Peter," an 8-year-old in treatment for phonological delay, who expresses the loss of trust when describing how the clinician did not follow-up on a promise:

My worst day going [to speech and language therapy], was when she promised me to have these pencils I liked, like she said she had them for me, she promised and then when I went she never had them there. She forgot an awful lot of times. (p. 318)

Also emerging as a theme is the role of routine and ritual in the children's life-world experiences of therapy. All of the children in the study describe the therapeutic process in terms of the routines and rituals in which they engaged with the clinician. The importance of these elements, according to the authors, is that they represent the nature of the rapport between the child and the clinician. Again, this is illustrated in the following descriptions provided by "Mary," another 8-year-old with phonological delay:

> If I get [pronunciation] right she gives me a sticker, and if I get another right she gives me two stickers, and another right she gives me more stickers. I like getting stickers. . . . She [clinician] was really nice. She thought I was a Super-girl. We used to pretend. She went out and then she'd come back in and she'd be like "Where did you go? Supergirl disappeared with her super powers." (p. 318)

Fourie et al. (2011) refer to "role confusion" as another element in the therapeutic relationship. Specifically, some of the children demonstrated confusion as to the particular role the SLP had in their education. For example, several of the children conceptualized the SLP as a teacher and therefore expected the therapist to teach subjects, such as reading or math, or they referred to the work of therapy in terms similar to that of school work. Finally, the physical characteristics of the clinician present themselves as factors in two of the children's comments. Overall, Fourie et al. conclude that children describe therapy in positive terms, although they might not always be able to articulate its purpose. With respect to making measurable gains in therapy, it is vital that the child and her or his family have an understanding of treatment goals and tasks. This is best achieved through a partnership or collaboration with all involved. By determining the most appropriate goals and crafting tasks to address those goals together with the child and family, trust is built and the therapeutic alliance is fortified.

A Reflection Exercise on the Therapeutic Alliance
Watch the Jen video from our library. First, jot down your thoughts on the client, then do so for the clinician. Keeping in mind the features of a therapeutic alliance, what behaviors do you see the client using to move the relationship forward? What behaviors do you see the clinician using to move the relationship forward? What is your reaction to what you have observed—cognitively and affectively?

A Note About the ICF and the Therapeutic Alliance

How do the ICF and its Child and Youth frameworks (ICF-CY) dovetail with the provision of audiology and speech-language pathology services? If we remember, the construct of *Impairment–Disability–Handicap* is used by the ICF to characterize the nature and impact of such impairments as hearing loss. An audiogram showing both air and bone conduction thresholds at above 70 dB for the frequency range of 250 to 8,000 Hz is evidence of an *impairment* in hearing sensitivity. Such an impairment might result in difficulty with speech perception or sound localization, which would be considered examples of *disability*. The *handicap* from such circumstances represents the impact they have on daily life, the nonauditory effects. An example of handicap might be the difficulties someone has using a telephone to accomplish a myriad of tasks.

In addition to the impact of the disability on the individual, the ICF also characterizes "third-party" disability as a disability experienced by someone within the affected individual's significant others or family as a result of their family member's disability. As an example, a systematic review of literature on the effects of living with and supporting an individual with aphasia reveals diverse outcomes in all realms of the ICF (Grawburg, Howe, Worrall, & Scarinci, 2013). That is, family members and those close to individuals with aphasia experience a multiplicity of effects and disabilities related to body functions, activities, and participation. Whereas some of these effects are positive, most include some type of negative impact. Families report difficulties with worry, which can impact sleeping patterns and energy level. Also reported are adjustments/restrictions in daily life, such as additional tasks taken on by family members, alterations in diet or meal planning, and considerable changes in communication and social activities. We are reminded that a communication impairment likely has wide-ranging implications for many people, not just the individual. Thus, any application of the ICF must respect the whole of individuals and their communities within which they interact.

Travis Threats (2010), an SLP and researcher who has conducted work on the application of the ICF to speech-language pathology, explains that the World Health Organization's (WHO's) philosophy defines health as ". . . the state of complete physical, mental, and social well-being" and ". . . communication as part of one's mental and social well-being" (p. 51). The tenets of the ICF are that it regards the individual as a full participant and the center of the health care process. Any assessment of behaviors using the ICF framework uses a holistic orientation (as we have been advocating for throughout this text), places them in appropriate contexts, and has ethical implications (Threats, 2010). There are several ethical considerations organized around three primary areas: (1) respect and confidentiality, (2) clinical use of the ICF, and (3) social use of ICF information (outlined by the WHO, 2001, pp. 244–245). It is important for audiologists and SLPs to be familiar with these guidelines in order to fully position themselves in ethically and morally sound practice. Respect and confidentiality are about having the highest regard for and valuing the person, regardless of disability or particular characteristics. The professional who truly respects the client/patient will include her or him and important others in all aspects of the therapeutic process. This involves more than simply sharing the results of an assessment or asking the individual what she or he would like to do that day. It means respecting the individual at all times, even when not engaged with her or him. Confidentiality is enactment of that respect, being sure to view the client/

patient respectfully, even when she or he is not present. The clinical use of the ICF refers to how one includes *all* aspects of the framework, including the environmental and personal factors along with the body structure and function components. These are the contextual aspects—the where, when, and how, the essence of our client's/patient's communication. The third element of ethical consideration is the social use of the ICF. In some ways, this is when we not only "talk the talk," we also "walk the walk." Our clients/patients are functioning human beings with real lives to live and it is our job to help them in doing just that. As Threats (2010) states:

> Society has no "spare" people. The child who stutters severely may be brilliant in physics and able to contribute to our understanding of our world, but will not be able to realize this societal contribution if not fully valued. The child who has trouble learning to read because of phonological processing difficulties may turn out to be an award winning artist whose works move persons to action. The adult who has had a stroke and aphasia may still be able to talk to grandchild [*sic*] who is severely depressed and help him or her feel she has a reason to live. The adult with severe dysarthria can still teach another person how to fix a broken car. (p. 92)

In their recent review of the literature related to measuring outcomes of preschoolers in speech and language therapy, Cunningham et al. (2017) note that SLPs adequately address participation-based concerns in therapy and they are successful at measuring outcomes relative to activities and body functions within the ICF-CY framework. However, during assessment, the evaluation of participation is often overlooked. These authors remind us that,

> Within the ICF-CF framework, a child's functioning and disability are viewed as being in dynamic interaction between health conditions and contextual factors. For instance, an impairment at the level of the body functions and structures, such as a speech sound disorder, influences not only the child's speech sound system, but also the child's ability to perform Activities (e.g., reading) as well as to Participate (e.g., engage in peer interactions; WHO, 2007). (p. 2)

Gagné, Jennings, and Southall (2014) highlight the usefulness in applying the ICF framework to issues of hearing, in particular to audiologic rehabilitation. Notably, the ICF provides a way to describe the functional impacts of hearing loss on both the individual with the impairment and others with normal hearing who interact with the person with hearing loss. These authors point out that clients/patients themselves can be guided by an audiologist using the ICF in a discussion of the limitations the hearing impairment places on the individual and her or his interactants. Thus, the application of the ICF model provides valuable information on the impact of the hearing loss and facilitates the development of a treatment program that will address the individual's specific concerns and those of the people with whom they interact. Gagné et al. declare,

Two important points about using the ICF to identify the goals of a rehabilitation program are that: (1) They necessarily involve the person consulting in the process of identifying the goals of rehabilitation as this person is best qualified to identify the most important activity limitations/participation restrictions they experience; and (2) the rehabilitation program, and more specifically the goals of the rehabilitation program, will be formulated in functional terms . . . (p. 51)

We can visualize these interactions by returning to the ICF descriptions provided in Chapter 2 in Tables 2–5 and 2–6. We see that Activities and Participation are impacted by environmental and personal factors. Again, these represent contextual factors that are essential to consider when planning and implementing communication assessment and intervention. Howe (2008) provides a summary of these factors as related to speech-language pathology, but they are equally applicable to audiology. She states three reasons why it is important to integrate environmental and personal factors into speech and language therapy (audiological services/rehabilitation). The first one is that expectations for clients and patients include using their communication in activities and participating in communicative situations outside the space in which therapy takes place. The second reason is that communication naturally involves social interaction and must take place with others. Those "others" are considered "environmental factors." And the third reason is that the SLP and audiologist possess the knowledge to assess the role environmental factors play in communication disorders. When it comes to environmental factors related to communication and its impairment, there are several components to consider, such as technology, sound or visual distractions, supports for the person with communication impairment, available services and policies, as well as attitudes regarding communication disorders. Personal factors are those characteristics associated with the individual that are not a result of or causative to the person's health condition. Some have suggested that personal factors be categorized into features that cannot be changed or are difficult to change (e.g., age, gender, ethnicity, and socioeconomic status) and those that can be altered (e.g., other health status, coping style, education, psychological assets; Howe, 2008). Personality and environmental factors are likely to interact as well. For instance, an individual with an outgoing personality who has a hearing loss may have greater success with making lifestyle changes that preserve ongoing social relationships than someone who is more reserved. The audiologist or SLP has an obligation to her or his clients/patients to evaluate these types of factors as they relate to facilitating or hindering communication and work with the client/patient to address them in treatment.

It is important to recognize that not all audiologists and SLPs have embraced the ICF framework. Duchan (2004) asks, "How can clinicians nowadays, make sure to find and support the person hidden behind the objectively assigned code or objectifying diagnosis" (p. 64)? Duchan's concern lies in the temptation to focus on the ICF codes for determining the effects of the communication impairment while neglecting that our interest lies with the client/patient as she or he functions in the world. She proposes the use of narrative discourse to reveal the story behind the disorder, stating, "Personal narratives are, for many, the best means to convey and understand a person's life experiences" (p. 64). As mentioned earlier, narratives have been incorporated into medical practice for some time. Its use represents moving beyond the "surface features" and learning about the client/patient in her or his own words. By taking the time to listen to their story, we gain invaluable insight. Fourie et al. (2011) stress the value of the "phenomenological" approach to learning about how the person's participation in the world is impacted by communication impairment. Phenomenology is the study of experience—what is the client's/patient's experience. Getting the person's story should be as critical to the diagnostic process as are formal and standardized measures. The narrative fits well within the ICF framework. Thus, as long as we do not see the ICF as a way of categorizing clients/patients as ". . . objects to code rather than human beings to support," Duchan articulates, ". . . speech-language pathologists can use the ICF to argue for a broader view of communication, one that has more to do with life participation and engagement than sending and receiving messages" (p. 65).

Overall, the ICF is much too large a document and its process too involved to teach within this text. However, it embodies a means by which we can come to understand our clients/patients, their loved ones, and their world experiences. But, as Threats expresses in his address to the Speech Pathology Australia National Conference in 2009,

> The ICF can be an effective tool to reach our field's general aspiration for optimum functioning of all persons with communication disorders. However, the ICF is a thing. A thing can contain written aspirations, just as a constitution for a country does. But aspiration is a human trait, something that has to be felt. Printed words on a page can only be inspiration if there is a human receiver who is so moved. Thus, the ICF can be a practical tool to achieve the highest vision of full integration of persons with functional health limitations in society, but only if that is what people decide they want. Individual speech-language pathologists must decide whether they view their job as just a job. The higher view of the field is for us to be part of the greatest of all humankind's aspiration—to all join as one, equal and together. (Threats, 2010, p. 92)

Clinically Significant Change

A final note about the therapeutic alliance is that of its association with "clinically significant change." The notion of clinically significant change may reflect different things depending on who is assessing the meaningfulness of any change observed. For example, clients may see any movement toward a goal (or away from a behavior deemed unacceptable) as significant, whereas a clinician may see clinically significant change as simply the reduction of an undesirable behavior and/or the increase of a desirable behavior. Manning (2010) points out, however, that this dichotomy may not be applicable in all therapeutic contexts.

For example, in stuttering therapy, whereas the clinician may see the reduction in overt stuttering behavior as clinically significant, the client may recognize it as the use of unacceptable behaviors, such as word substitutions, to hide the stuttering. This is illustrated in a quote borrowed by Manning (2010) from Plexico, Manning, and Levitt (2009):

> When I was in therapy in junior high I would substitute and I would not stutter and she [speech therapist] would think that I was making progress, but I was hiding it the whole time. I don't know why I would hide it from the speech pathologist you know, but it was just that I was ashamed of it, so any chance I could dodge a block I took it. So she thought I was making so much progress. (p. 209)

Before tackling this question, it is important we understand what is meant by meaningful or clinically significant change. In order to establish that such change has occurred in the context of treatment, Bain and Dollaghan (1991) argue that three criteria must be met:

> A clinically significant change is a change in client performance that (a) can be shown to result from treatment rather than from maturation or other uncontrolled factors, (b) can be shown to be real, rather than random, and (c) can be shown to be important, rather than trivial. (p. 265)

These authors point out that clinicians in the "real world" can establish that change is occurring because of treatment by collecting data, over time, on target behaviors in comparison to behaviors not being targeted in therapy. If improvement is observed in the treated behaviors and not the comparison behaviors, one has documented change that is due directly to therapy. To verify that change is real, Bain and Dollaghan suggest ". . . the best evidence . . . comes from careful measurements of the change with valid and reliable instruments" (p. 266). A valid measure is one that truly assesses the behavior of interest, whereas a reliable measure is one that is consistent in its measurement, regardless when it is used or by whom. This process is not one of simply readministering the same test but involves the use of measurements and instruments that may be designed by the clinician. As an example, the clinician can set a criterion of the number or percentage of correct productions of a sound in a particular context for a child to achieve in order to measure that child's progress. A master clinician also will review the literature for other examples of valid and reliable ways to document progress or check in with colleagues as a means of confirming the validity of her/his chosen measurement. The third component included in the notion of "clinically significant change" is that of the importance of the change. This can be conceptualized as significant change as demonstrated by a score on an appropriate test or instrument that has adequate psychometric properties or by its impact on the client/patient. When using standardized measures with applicable normative information, the clinician must take into consideration the size of the change in score observed. In other words, using test standard scores and comparing those to what is expected for typical speakers, a clinician can determine how far from typical her or his client's/patient's performance falls at the beginning of treatment and at some point after the client/patient has been receiving therapy. If the change is large (a standard deviation or more), the clinician can be assured the change is significant. Examples of this procedure are explained in Bain and Dollaghan and Friel-Patti, DesBarres, and Thibodeau (2001). Using observer, client/patient, or family member ratings or perceptions regarding the change that has happened is another valuable way of determining the importance of the change. This approach, it has been argued, is the only "real" way to determine if treatment is making a difference (Kazdin, 2003).

Overall, an examination of clinically significant change from the client's/patient's/family member's perspectives may be the only factor that truly matters in the therapeutic process. It is not my intention to argue that we should not be using standard measures to track progress. Certainly, technical/clinical measures are necessary for documenting change for all kinds of reasons (e.g., to satisfy third-party payers, to maintain clinical records, and to provide "hard evidence" to other professionals). However, when it comes down to the daily lives of our clients/patients, it may not always be clear (based on traditional methods of assessing significant change) that we are effecting meaningful change (Kazdin, 2003). As Kazdin's (2003) work reminds us, the process of change often takes place in small, less conspicuous steps, and these smaller movements may have substantial effects on the client's/patient's perspective on therapy and change. Although specific to stuttering, Manning's (2010) commentary on meaningful change pertains to all of speech and language therapy. He describes elements related to the change process that are important to consider. The first of these is the idea of stages of change. According to Manning,

> Studies in psychology and counseling have demonstrated that the utility of the techniques used in treatment often depends on the clinician's ability to apply the right therapeutic technique(s), or process at the right time. We also have to have the wisdom *not* to use a particular technique if the timing is not appropriate. (p. 209, italics in original)

Much like Goldberg's "exquisite timing," a clinician and client working toward meaningful change must recognize the stage at which the client is relative to readiness for change and make clinical decisions with this in mind.

In their discussion of theories of change and planned behavior related to stuttering treatment in adolescents, Floyd, Zebrowski, and Flamme (2007) note that, initially, a client/patient must have an intention to change, which is based on three aspects: (1) how acceptable/unacceptable the behavior is to her or him; (2) how acceptable/unacceptable the behavior is to others; and (3) self-efficacy, or how likely it is the person will be successful in making change. In the therapeutic process, these factors influence how ready the client is to start on the path to change. The path to change has been described in stages (Prochaska & DiClemente, 1984), which include *precontemplation, contemplation, preparation, action,* and *maintenance.* In precontemplation, feelings about oneself are explored; contemplation involves collecting information about the issue and how to address it as well as continuing to assess oneself; preparation often involves some type of decision to act; action includes making conscious choices to do things differently and gain support from others; and maintenance is ongoing action, beliefs, and rewarding oneself for changes made. From a speech and language therapy perspective, the clinician must take into account the stage at which the client/patient is in terms of change, and the types of processes the client/patient might be ready to use in moving toward change. As described by Prochaska and DiClemente (1984), movement toward change takes place at different levels of complexity. For the practitioner in speech and language therapy, this might include tasks early on that are considered less complex and likely to result in change more quickly. An example from stuttering therapy might be direct work on specific speaking techniques that modify the stuttering or facilitate fluent speech (Floyd et al., 2007). As the client moves along in the change process, openness to and need for more complex activities will become germane. Thus, a clinician working with a client regarding speech fluency might introduce tasks in which the client is expected to reflect on her or his own performance or the effects of different external factors on communication success.

A second factor Manning (2010) associates with change is the client's/patient's manner in which she or he copes. Coping involves the use of strategies, cognitive and behavioral, to manage circumstances that are considered to exert demands that go beyond an individual's capacities (Lazarus & Folkman, 1984). These strategies have been conceptualized as emotion based or cognitive based (Manning, 2010). With emotion-based forms of coping, behaviors are exhibited that are designed to avoid or reduce discomfort. Manning notes that these could include ". . . avoidance, minimizing, distancing, selective attention, positive comparison, and finding positive value in negative events" (p. 210). Cognitive-based strategies include efforts to reduce or eliminate the effects of something threatening. These types of responses are employed in circumstances where the person believes she or he can do something to address the threat. According to Manning, cognitive-based coping includes ". . . defining the problem, generating alternative solutions, weighing alternatives in terms of cost and benefit, and choosing among multiple solutions" (p. 210). Recent research on coping in clients/patients with communication impairment includes a study by Plexico et al. (2009), which explored coping strategies used by adults who stutter. The upshot of this work is that individuals who stutter perceive the experience of stuttering as very stressful and they employ both cognitive-based and emotion-based strategies in attempting to deal with the threat of stuttering. What these authors and Manning observe is that cognitive-based responses to the threat of stuttering allow clients to develop greater self-efficacy in terms of how they might cope with stuttering. Rather than avoiding the possibility of stuttering, clients who use cognitive-based coping strategies considered themselves first (as opposed to the listener) and adopt approach behaviors. The implications of this work are that

".... clinicians need to understand and appreciate the core belief system of their clients and how clients' belief systems are shaping their coping choices. .... it may also be wise for us to focus on assisting clients in becoming mindful of their current situation and alternative solutions to coping . . ." (Plexico et al., 2009, p. 104)

So, with a goal of helping clients/patients make meaningful change through the various stages and the development of positive coping behaviors, where does the therapeutic alliance come in? The connection involves making certain we embrace the client's/patient's perspectives on change, the therapy process, and how well the alliance is working. We need to make routine the use of scales, questionnaires, and other mechanisms for garnering client/patient feedback. Given what we know about the substantial effect of the therapeutic alliance on treatment outcomes, it makes sense to routinely collect feedback on the relationship from our clients/patients. Brown, Cameron, and Brown (2008), psychologists and researchers with expertise in the use of data (i.e., client/patient feedback) to improve outcomes, underscore the importance of the interaction between outcomes and the therapeutic relationship:

In an era of increasing demands that treatments of all kinds be "proven effective" it is important not to lose sight of the simple fact that all treatments involve a relationship between a human being in need and a helping professional. This includes the relationship between a speech-language pathologist and a client . . . speech-language pathologists might want to be increasingly sensitive to their relationships with clients and do everything they can to promote a therapeutic alliance. (pp. 57–58)

Chapter Summary

In summary, we explore aspects of the therapeutic relationship, sometimes referred to as the therapeutic alliance, in mental health, allied health, and the CSD discipline. In large measure, the effectiveness of intervention can be traced to the strength of the relationship between the practitioner and patient/client and the alliance formed between them as they work toward mutual goals. We have learned that, without a partnership, therapeutic progress is jeopardized. Emphasis is placed on using narrative processes to facilitate mutual understanding and co-construction of a therapeutic alliance. The issue of meaningful change is introduced, with the suggestion that practitioners and clients/patients may have very different perspectives on what constitutes meaningful change. Again, the formulation of an effective therapeutic process takes place through the course of establishing a positive working alliance, something that is facilitated by integrating client/patient perspective with clinician expertise. The reader is invited to contemplate what "change" means to her or him.

For the student and beginning clinician, experience with listening to and appreciating people's stories will go a long way toward the development of skills necessary for establishing alliances with future clients and patients. In observing clinical interactions, we can work to determine if a positive therapeutic alliance is present. What behaviors on the part of the clinician tell you that she or he is using a model of alliance in therapy? What behaviors on the part of the client/patient reveal an understanding and acceptance of the goals and tasks of treatment and the bond with the clinician? Imagine yourself as the clinician— what skills could you rely on to facilitate developing a therapeutic relationship with a client or patient?

Chapter Observations and Exercises

Exercise 5-1: Observing the Therapeutic Relationship

Watch the "KD" video; what strategies do you see the clinician using to establish therapeutic change? What effects do they have?

Exercise 5-2: Clinician Interview

For this exercise, you will conduct an interview with a practicing audiologist or SLP. The purpose of the interview is to learn how the clinician perceives the therapeutic relationship and what strategies or techniques she or he relies on to establish and maintain the alliance. Describe this purpose to the practitioner; explain that it is an assignment for your class (identify the class and university) and that you will be asking only a few questions. Explain how you will be collecting the answers (i.e., recording, writing, etc.; preferably you should be writing down your notes, rather than recording them), and you will be handing in a short paper summarizing the interview. You will not be sharing the person's name in the written assignment. Before proceeding, be sure to ask if she or he has any objection or questions. Pose your questions as such:

a. Are you familiar with the concept of a therapeutic alliance? How would you define it?
b. When establishing a working relationship with your clients or patients, what types of strategies or techniques do you use?

Assignment constraints and requirements:

- You may NOT interview any faculty or clinical supervisors within your academic program.
- Be sure you are polite in your interactions and express your thanks when finishing up the interview.
- Your write-up should be no more than two pages typed, double spaced, and include basic information about the person you interview (e.g., audiologist or SLP, years of professional experience), their work setting/practice characteristics (e.g., setting, typical populations working with), and if the interview was conducted in person or via telephone, Skype, etc.
- Include their responses to the questions, what you learned from the interview, and at least one aspect that surprised you.

Exercise 5-3: Eco-Mapping

Imagine you are the client/patient, and your clinician is engaging you in a process of eco-mapping. Draw out what your map might look like—who would be involved? What is the strength of the connections? Make some notes on your map related to the ways in which the various elements on the map might be helpful in therapy.

Exercise 5–4: Finding Resources for Involving Family Members

Imagine you are the clinician working with a client/patient whose family members are greatly involved in the therapeutic process. Do some research on available instruments for collecting input from family members or those significant to the client/patient. List at least three and identify what each might be best used for.

APPENDIX

Disability Memoirs and Stories

Listed below are several books, websites, podcasts, and others, on the experience of a disability. Most of these are true, nonfiction accounts from the individual's or family's perspective, although a few works of fiction are included. It is not an exhaustive list by any means, as there are many, many, many stories out there. I chose not to include blogs or websites of various organizations that might include personal stories or newsletters with stories because there are just too many. This list is here as a resource for learning more about the experience of living with a disability. I have used a number of the texts in my classes, and students almost always find they gain at least a little insight into the worlds of people living with disabilities on a daily basis. Often, students will have read books, seen movies, or explored online resources and shared them with me—some are included in the listing below. On occasion, I have required students to do their own research and come up with a list of memoirs they would recommend to other students. Our department has had a tradition of reading a series of texts in our senior capstone course and selecting a favorite to then be assigned to beginning students in the introductory communication sciences and disorders course. Perhaps your local student organization could start up a book club, or one of your instructors will choose to include a few of these resources with other classes. I encourage you to carve out some time and delve into a text or two—happy reading (or viewing or listening)!

Alzheimer's Disease

Alzheimer's Daughter—Jean Lee

A Cup of Comfort for Families Touched by Alzheimer's: Inspirational Stories of Unconditional Love and Support—Colleen Sell

Keeper: One House, Three Generations, and a Journey into Alzheimer's—Andrea Gillies

Losing My Mind: An Intimate Look at Life With Alzheimer's—Thomas DeBaggio

Still Alice—Lisa Genova

Tangles: A Story About Alzheimer's, My Mother, and Me—Sarah Leavitt

Autism

Asperger Syndrome in the Family—Liane Willey Holliday

Born on a Blue Day—Daniel Tammet

Carly's Voice: Breaking Through Autism—Arthur Fleischmann

The Curious Incident of the Dog in the Nighttime—Mark Haddon

Elijah's Cup—Valerie Paradiz

Emergence: Labelled Autistic—Temple Grandin

How Can I Talk if My Lips Don't Move: Inside My Autistic Mind—
Tito Rajarshi Mukhopadhyay

Making Peace With Autism—Susan Senator

Mixed Blessings—William and Barbara Christopher

Not Even Wrong—Paul Collins

Pretending to be Normal—Liane Willey Holliday

Raising Blaze—Debra Ginsberg

Thinking in Pictures—Temple Grandin

Without Reason: A Family Copes With Two Generations of Autism—
Charles Hart

Brain Injury/Neurological Impairment

The Day My Brain Exploded—Ashok Rajamani

The Defiant Mind: Living Inside a Stroke—Ron Smith

The Diving Bell and the Butterfly—Jean-Dominque Baury

Head Cases: Stories of Brain Injury and Its Aftermath—Michael
Paul Mason

*I Remember Running: The Year I Got Everything I Wanted—And
ALS*—Darcy Wakefield

Left Neglected—Lisa Genova

My Stroke of Insight: A Brain Scientist's Personal Journey—Jill Bolte
Taylor

One Hundred Names for Love: A Stroke, a Marriage, and the Language of Healing—Diane Ackerman

Tuesdays With Morrie—Mitch Albom

Where Is the Mango Princess?—Cathy Crimmins

Deafness/Hearing Loss

Alone in the Mainstream—Gina Oliva

Finding Zoe: A Deaf Woman's Story of Identity, Love and Adoption—Brandi Rarus and Gail Harris

If You Could Hear What I See: Triumph Over Tragedy Through Laughter—Kathy Buckley

Like Sound through Water—Karen J. Foli

Seeing Voices: A Journey into the World of the Deaf—Oliver Sacks

Train Go Sorry: Inside a Deaf World—Leah Hager Cohen

What's That Pig Outdoors?—Henry Kisor

Down Syndrome/Developmental Disability

Count Us In: Growing Up With Down Syndrome—Jason Kingsley and Mitchell Levitz

Expecting Adam—Martha Beck

Gifts: Mothers Reflect on How Children With Down Syndrome Enrich Their Lives—Kathryn Lynard Soper

Life With Charley: A Memoir of Down Syndrome Adoption—Sherry McCalley Palmer

My Baby Rides the Short Bus: The Unabashedly Human Experience of Raising Kids With Disabilities—Yantra Bertelli

Riding the Bus With My Sister—Rachel Simon

Learning Disability

A Different Life: Growing Up Learning Disabled and Other Adventures—Quinn Bradley and Jeff Himmelman

Laughing Allegra—Anne Ford

Learning Disabilities and Life Stories—Pano Rodis

Legacy of the Blue Heron: Living With Learning Disabilities—Harry Sylvester

Speech and Language Disorder

BEING SPECIAL: A Mother and Son's Journey With Speech Disorders and Learning Disabilities—Barbara L. Curry and David Curry

Kids Speech Matters: A Mother's Journey Living With Her Son Who Has a Severe Language and Auditory Processing Disorder—Sandra Ahlquist

Stuttering

Forty Years After Therapy: One Man's Story—George G. Helliensen

The King's Speech—Mark Logue and Peter Conradi

Knotted Tongues—Benson Bobrick

Living With Stuttering: Stories, Basics, Resources and Hope—Kenneth O. St. Louis

Out With It: How Stuttering Helped Me Find My Voice—Katherine Preston

Stutter—Marc Shell

A Stutterer's Story—Frederick Pemberton Murray

Voice: A Stutterer's Odyssey—Scott Damian

Other

Don't Worry, He Won't Get Far on Foot—John Callahan

Far From the Tree—Andrew Solomon

A Leg to Stand On—Oliver Sacks

The Man Who Mistook His Wife for a Hat—Oliver Sacks

Moving Violations: Way Zones, Wheelchairs, and Declarations of Independence—John Hockenberry

Robyn's Book—Robyn Miller

Wheels for Walking—Sandra Richmond

The World I Live In—Helen Keller

Ted Talks

Title: How Autism Freed Me to Be Myself

Category: Autism

Link: https://www.ted.com/talks/rosie_king_how_autism_freed_me_to
_be_myself

Description: "People are so afraid of variety that they try to fit everything into a tiny little box with a specific label," says 16-year-old Rosie
King, who is bold, brash, and autistic. She wants to know: Why is
everyone so worried about being normal? She sounds a clarion call
for every kid, parent, teacher, and person to celebrate uniqueness. It's
a soaring testament to the potential of human diversity.

Title: Matthew Williams: Special Olympics Let Me Be Myself—
A Champion

Category: Intellectual disability

Link: https://www.ted.com/talks/matthew_williams_special_olympics
_let_me_be_myself_a_champion

Description: How much do you know about intellectual disabilities?
Special Olympics champion and ambassador Matthew Williams is
proof that athletic competition and the camaraderie it fosters can
transform lives, both on and off the field. Together with his fellow
athletes, he invites you to join him at the next meet—and challenges
you to walk away with your heart unchanged.

Title: I Got 99 Problems . . . Palsy Is Just One

Category: Cerebral palsy

Link: http://www.ted.com/talks/maysoon_zayid_i_got_99_problems
_palsy_is_just_one

Description: "I have cerebral palsy. I shake all the time," Maysoon
Zayid announces at the beginning of this exhilarating, hilarious talk.
(Really, it's hilarious.) "I'm like Shakira meets Muhammad Ali." With
grace and wit, the Arab-American comedian takes us on a whistle-stop
tour of her adventures as an actress, stand-up comic, philanthropist,
and advocate for the disabled.

Title: How Technology Allowed Me to Read

Category: Blind

Link: https://www.ted.com/talks/ron_mccallum_how_technology
_allowed_me_to_read#t-136553

Description: Months after he was born, in 1948, Ron McCallum became blind. In this charming, moving talk, he shows how he reads—and celebrates the progression of clever tools and adaptive computer technologies that make it possible. With their help, and the help of volunteers, he's become a lawyer, an academic, and most of all, a voracious reader. Welcome to the blind reading revolution.

Title: In the Key of Genius

Category: Autism/Blind/Premature Birth

Link: https://www.ted.com/talks/derek_paravicini_and_adam_ockelford_in_the_key_of_genius

Description: Born three and a half months prematurely, Derek Paravicini is blind and has severe autism. But with perfect pitch, innate talent, and a lot of practice, he became a concert pianist by the age of 10. Here, his longtime piano teacher, Adam Ockelford, explains his student's unique relationship to music, while Paravicini shows how he has ripped up the "Chopsticks" rulebook.

Title: Embrace the Shake

Category: Tremor

Link: https://www.ted.com/talks/phil_hansen_embrace_the_shake

Description: In art school, Phil Hansen developed an unruly tremor in his hand that kept him from creating the pointillist drawings he loved. Hansen was devastated, floating without a sense of purpose. Until a neurologist made a simple suggestion: embrace this limitation . . . and transcend it.

Title: Deaf in the Military

Category: Deaf

Link: https://www.ted.com/talks/keith_nolan_deaf_in_the_military

Description: Keith Nolan always wanted to join the U.S. military. The challenge: He is deaf, which is an automatic disqualification according to military rules. In this talk, he describes his fight to fight for his country. (In American Sign Language, with real-time translation.)

Title: Looking Past Limits

Category: Ocular Albinism (vision)

Link: https://www.ted.com/talks/caroline_casey_looking_past_limits

Description: Activist Caroline Casey tells the story of her extraordinary life, starting with a revelation (no spoilers). In a talk that challenges perceptions, Casey asks us all to move beyond the limits we may think we have.

Title: My 12 Pairs of Legs

Category: Amputee

Link: https://www.ted.com/talks/aimee_mullins_prosthetic_aesthetics

Description: Athlete, actor, and activist Aimee Mullins talks about her prosthetic legs—she's got a dozen amazing pairs—and the superpowers they grant her: speed, beauty, an extra 6 inches of height. . . . Quite simply, she redefines what the body can be.

Podcasts

Title: Ouch: Disability Talk

Category: Various

Link: Podcast

Description: Interviews and discussion with a personal and often humorous touch. With guest presenters plus Katie Monaghan and the Ouch blog team. Ouch is available exclusively online and goes out every week.

Title: Disability Matters

Category: Various

Link: Podcast

Description: Competitive employment and empowerment for people with disabilities are the emphases of this show. Broadcast live and captioned in real-time for individuals who are deaf and hard of hearing, we discuss how people with disabilities can secure career opportunities and how employers, organizations, and individuals can support employment and empowerment of people with disabilities.

Title: StutterTalk

Category: Stuttering

Link: http://stuttertalk.com

Description: StutterTalk is a 501 (c)(3) nonprofit organization dedicated to talking openly about stuttering. StutterTalk is the first and longest running podcast on stuttering. Since 2007, we have published more than 600 podcasts. StutterTalk is heard in more than 170 countries.

REFERENCES

Abrami, P. C., Bernard, R. M., Borokhovski, E., Wade, A., Surkes, M. A., Tamim, R., & Zhang, D. (2008). Instructional interventions affecting critical thinking skills and dispositions: A Stage I meta-analysis. *Review of Educational Research, 78,* 1102–1134.

Adamson, B. J., Hand, L. S., Heard, R., & Nordholm, L. A. (1999). Australian speech pathologists' views of what professional practices lead to successful outcomes of therapy. *Journal of Allied Health, 28,* 137–147.

American Speech-Language-Hearing Association. (1995, March). Position statement: Facilitated communication. *Asha, 37* (Suppl. 14), 22.

American Speech-Language-Hearing Association. (2004). *Scope of Practice in Audiology.* [Scope of Practice]. Available from http://www.asha.org/policy/SP2004 -00192.htm.

American Speech-Language-Hearing Association. (2015). *The role of undergraduate education in communication sciences and disorders.* Rockville, MD: Author.

American Speech-Language-Hearing Association. (2016a). *Standards for accreditation for graduate programs in audiology and speech-language pathology (Effective August 1, 2017).* Rockville, MD: ASHA.

American Speech-Language-Hearing Association. (2016b). *Scope of practice in speech-language pathology* [scope of practice]. Available from http://www.asha.org/policy /SP2016-00343/.

Anderson, D. K., Liang, J. W., & Lord, C. (2014). Predicting young adult outcome among more and less cognitively able individuals with autism spectrum disorders. *Journal of Child Psychology and Psychiatry, 55,* 485–494.

Anderson, T., Ogles, B. M., Patterson, D. L., Lambert, M. J., & Vermeersch, D. A. (2009). Therapist effects: Facilitative interpersonal skills as a predictor of therapist success. *Journal of Clinical Psychology, 65,* 755–768.

Ashby, S. B., Adler, J., & Herbert, L. (2016). An exploratory international study of occupational therapy students' perceptions of professional identity. *Australian Occupational Therapy Journal, 63,* 233–243.

Bain, B. A., & Dollaghan, C. A. (1991). Treatment efficacy: The notion of clinically significant change. *Language, Speech, Hearing Services in Schools, 22,* 264–270.

Baldwin, S. A., & Imel, Z. E. (2013). Therapist effects: Findings and methods. In M. J. Lambert (Ed.), *Bergin and Garfield's handbook of psychotherapy and behavior change* (pp. 258–297). Hoboken, NJ: John Wiley & Sons.

Baldwin, S. A., Wampold, B. E., & Imel, Z. E. (2007). Untangling the alliance-outcome connection: Exploring the relative importance of therapist and patient variability in the alliance. *Journal of Consulting Clinical Psychology, 75,* 842–852.

Barnett, R. (1997). *Higher education: A critical business.* Buckingham, England: The Society for Research into Higher Education and Open University Press.

Batson, C. D. (1998). Altruism and prosocial behavior. In D. T. Gilbert, S. T. Fiske, & G. Lindzey (Eds.), *The handbook of social psychology* (No. 2, pp. 282–316). New York, NY: McGraw-Hill.

Baxter, S. K., & Gray, C. (2001). The application of student-centred learning approaches to clinical learning. *International Journal of Language and Communication Disorders, 36*, 396–400.

Bendapudi, N. M., Berry, L. L., Frey, K. A., Turner Parish, J., & Rayburn, W. L. (2006). Patients' perspectives on ideal physician behaviors. *Mayo Clinic Proceedings, 81*, 338–344.

Berg, A. L., Canellas, M., Salbod, S., & Velayo, R. (2008). Exposure to disability and hearing loss narratives in undergraduate audiology curriculum. *American Journal of Audiology, 17*, 123–128.

Berger, L. R. (1980). Commentaries: A hierarchy of observations. *Pediatrics, 65*, 357–358.

Biklen, D. (1992). Typing to talk: Facilitated communication. *American Journal of Speech-Language Pathology, 1*, 15–17. doi:10.1044/1058-0360.0102.15

Black, L. L., Jensen, G. M., Mostrom, E., Perkins, J., Ritzline, P. D., Hayward, L., & Blackmer, B. (2010). The first year of practice: An investigation of the professional learning and development of promising novice physical therapists. *Physical Therapy, 90*, 1758–1773.

Blaire, I. (2002). The malleability of automatic stereotypes and prejudice. *Personality and Social Psychology Review, 6*, 247–261.

Bohart, A. C., & Greaves Wade, A. (2013). The client in psychotherapy. M. J. Lambert (Ed.). *Bergin and Garfield's handbook of psychotherapy and behavior change* (6th ed.) (pp. 219–257). Hoboken, NJ: John Wiley & Sons.

Bombeke, K., Symons, L., Vermeire, E., Debaene, L., Schol, S., De Winter, B., & Van Royen, P. (2012). Patient-centredness from education to practice: The 'lived' impact of communication skills training. *Medical Teacher, 34*, e338–e348.

Bombeke, K., Van Roosbroeck, S., De Winter, B., Debaene, L., Schol, S., Van Hal, G., & Van Royen, P. (2011). Medical students trained in communication skills show a decline in patient-centred attitudes: An observational study comparing two cohorts during clinical clerkships. *Patient Education and Counseling, 84*, 310–318.

Bordin, E. S. (1979). The generalizability of the psychoanalytic concept of the working alliance. *Psychotherapy: Theory, research, and practice, 16*, 252–260.

Boss, E., Niparko, J., Gaskin, D., & Levinson, K. (2011) Socioeconomic disparities for hearing-impaired children in the United States. *The Laryngoscope, 121*, 860–866.

Boud, D., Keogh, R., & Walker, D. (1985). *Reflection: Turning experience into learning*. London, England: Kogan Page.

Boudreau, J. D., Cassells, E. J., & Fuks, A. (2008). Preparing medical students to become skilled at clinical observation. *Medical Teacher, 30*, 857–862.

Bowman, D., Scogin, F., Floyd, M., & McKendree-Smith, N. (2001). Psychotherapy length of stay and outcome: A meta-analysis of the effect of therapist sex. *Psychotherapy: Theory, Research, Practice, Training, 38*, 142–148.

Braverman, I. M. (2011). To see or not to see: How visual training can improve observational skills. *Clinics in Dermatology, 29*, 343–346.

Brewer, M. B. (1988). A dual process model of impression formation. In T. K. Srull & R. S. Wyer (Eds.), *Advances in social cognition* (Vol. 1, pp. 1–36). Hillsdale, NJ: Lawrence Erlbaum Associates, Inc.

Brewer, M. B., & Brown, R. J. (1998). Intergroup relations. In D. T. Gilbert, S. T. Fiske, & J. Lindzey (Eds.), *The handbook of social psychology* (Vols. 1–2, 4th ed., pp. 554–594). Boston, MA: McGraw-Hill.

Brown, G. J., Cameron, J., & Brown, L. (2008). In search of the active ingredient: What really works in mental health care? *Perspectives on Fluency and Fluency Disorders, 18*, 53–59. doi:10.1044/ffd18.2.53

Brown, J. B., Thornton, T., & Stewart, M. (Eds.) (2012). *Challenges and solutions: Narratives of patient-centered care.* New York, NY: Radcliffe.

Browne, M. N., & Keeley, S. M. (2015). *Asking the right questions: A guide to critical thinking* (11th ed.). Upper Saddle River, NJ: Prentice Hall.

Budner, S. (1962). Intolerance of ambiguity as a personality variable. *Journal of Personality, 30*, 29–50.

Bulman, C., Lathlean, J., & Gobbi, M. (2012). The concept of reflection in nursing: Qualitative findings on student and teacher perspectives. *Nursing Education Today, 32*, e8–e13.

Burgess, D., van Ryn, M., Dovidio, J., Saha, S. (2007). Reducing racial bias among health care providers: Lessons from social cognitive psychology. *Journal of General Internal Medicine, 22*, 882–887.

Burns, M., Baylor, C., Dudgeon, B. J., Starks, H., & Yorkston, K. (2015). Asking the stakeholders: Perspectives of individuals with aphasia, their family members, and physicians regarding communication in medical interactions. *American Journal of Speech-Language Pathology, 24*, 341–357.

Campos, R. (2005). "The Medical Humanities," for lack of a better term (Reprinted). *Journal of the American Medical Association, 294*, 1009–1011.

Candlin, S. (2002). Taking risks: An indicator of expertise? *Research on Language and Social Interaction, 35*, 173–193.

Carey, E. T., & Miller, B. A. (2011, November). Developing a professional identity: One graduate student's experience. Presented to the *Annual Convention of the American Speech-Language-Hearing Association*, San Diego, CA.

Castonguay, L. G., & Beutler, L. E. (2006a). Common and unique principles of therapeutic change: What do we know and what do we need to know? In L. G. Castonguay & L. E. Beutler (Eds.), *Principles of therapeutic change that work* (pp. 353–370). New York, NY: Oxford University Press.

Castonguay, L. G., & Beutler, L. E. (2006b). *Principles of therapeutic change that work* (pp. 353–370). New York, NY: Oxford University Press.

Caty, M.-E., Kinsella, E. A., & Doyle, P. C. (2015). Reflective practice in speech-pathology: A scoping review. *International Journal of Speech-Language Pathology, 17*, 411–420.

Caughter, S., & Dunsmuir, S. (2017). An exploration of the mechanisms of change following an integrated group intervention for stuttering, as perceived by school-aged children who stutter. *Journal of Fluency Disorders, 51*, 8–23.

Caulfield, M., Andolsek, K., Grbic, D., & Roskovensky, L. (2014). Ambiguity tolerance of students matriculating to U.S. medical schools. *Academic Medicine, 89*, 1526–1532.

Charlton, C. R., Dearing, K. S., Berry, J. A., & Johnson, M. J. (2008). Nurse practitioners' communication styles and their impact on patient outcomes: An integrated literature review. *Journal of the American Academy of Nurse Practitioners, 20*, 383–388.

Charon, R. (2006). *Narrative medicine: Honoring the stories of illness.* New York, NY: Oxford University Press.

Chen, S.-L., Hsu, H.-Y., Chang, C.-F., & Lin, E. C.-L. (2016). An exploration of the correlates of nurse practitioners' clinical decision-making abilities. *Journal of Clinical Nursing, 25*, 1016–1025. doi:10.1111/jocn.13136

Ching, T. Y. C., & Dillon, H. (2013). Major findings of the LOCHI study on children at 3 years of age and implications for audiological management. *International Journal of Audiology, 52*, S65–S68.

Choi, D., Conture, E. G., Walden, T. A., Jones, R. M., & Kim, H. (2016). Emotional diathesis, emotional stress, and childhood stuttering. *Journal of Speech, Language, and Hearing Research, 59*, 616–630.

Cirrin, F. M., & Gillam, R. B. (2008). Language intervention practices for school-age children with spoken language disorders: A systematic review. *Language, Speech, and Hearing Services in Schools, 39*, S110–S137.

Clarke, N. M. (2014). A person-centred enquiry into the teaching and learning experiences of reflection and reflective practice—Part One. *Nurse Education Today, 34*, 1219–1224.

Clarkin, J. F., & Levy, K. N. (2004). The influence of client variables on psychotherapy. *Psychology and Psychotherapy: Theory, Research, and Practice, 77*, 67–89.

Cobelli, N., Gill, L., Cassia, F., & Ugolini, M. (2014). Factors that influence intent to adopt a hearing aid in older people in Italy. *Health and Social Care in the Community, 22*, 612–622. doi:10.1111/hsc.12127

Coles, R. (1979). Occasional notes. Medical ethics and living a life. *New England Journal of Medicine, 301*, 444–446.

Constantinou, M., & Kuys, S. S. (2013). Physiotherapy students find guided journals useful to develop reflective thinking and practice during their first clinical placement: A qualitative study. *Physiotherapy, 99*, 49–55.

Conway, S. (1998). Evolution of the species 'expert nurse.' An examination of the practical knowledge held by expert nurses. *Journal of Clinical Nursing, 7*, 75–82.

Cooke, D., Doust, J., & Steele, M. (2013). A survey of resilience, burnout, and intolerance of uncertainty in Australian general practice registrars. *BMC Medical Education, 13*, 2. doi:10.1186/1472-6920-13-2

Council for Clinical Certification in Audiology and Speech-Language Pathology of the American Speech-Language-Hearing Association. (2013). 2014 Standards for the Certificate of Clinical Competence in Speech-Language Pathology. Retrieved from http://www.asha.org/Certification/2014-Speech-Language-Pathology-Certification-Standards/.

Crandall, S. J., Reboussin, B. A., Michielutte, R., Anthony, J. E., & Naughton, M. J. (2007). Medical students' attitudes toward underserved patients: A longitudinal comparison of problem-based and traditional medical curricula. *Advances in Health Sciences Education, 12*, 71–86.

Crossley, R. (1992). Lending a hand: A personal account of the development of facilitated communication training. *American Journal of Speech-Language Pathology, 1*, 15–18.

Cruz, E. B., Caeiro, C., & Pareira, C. (2014). A narrative reasoning course to promote patient-centred practice in a physiotherapy undergraduate programme: A qualitative study of final year students. *Physiotherapy Theory and Practice, 30*, 254–260.

Cuijpers, P., van Straten, A., Smit, F., & Andersson, G. (2009). Is psychotherapy for depression equally effective for younger and older adults? A meta-regression analysis. *International Psychogeriatrics, 21*, 16–24.

Cunningham, B. J., Washington, K. N., Binns, A., Rolfe, K., Robertson, B., & Rosenbaum, P. (2017). Current methods of evaluating speech-language outcomes for preschoolers with communication disorders: A scoping review using the ICF-CY.

Journal of Speech, Language and Hearing Research. doi:10.1044/2016_JSLHR-L -15-0329

Daaleman, T. P., Kinghorn, W. A., Newton, W. P., & Meador, K. G. (2011). Rethinking professionalism in medical education through formation. *Family Medicine, 43,* 325–329.

Damico, J. S. (1993). Establishing expertise in communicative discourse: Implications for the speech-language pathologist. *ASHA Monographs, 30,* 92–98.

Danger, S., & Landreth, C. (2005). Child-centred group play therapy with children with speech difficulties. *International Journal of Play Therapy, 14,* 81–102.

De Vries, A. A. M., de Roten, Y., Meystre, C., Passchier, J., Despland, J.-N., & Stiefel, F. (2014). Clinician characteristics, communication, and patient outcome in oncology: A systematic review. *Psycho-Oncology, 23,* 375–381.

Del Re, A. C., Flückiger, C., Horvath, A. O., Symonds, D., & Wampold, B. E. (2012). Therapist effects in the therapeutic alliance-outcome relationship: A restricted-maximum likelihood meta-analysis. *Clinical Psychology Review, 32,* 642–649.

Deveugele, M. (2015). Communication skills: Training and beyond. *Patient Education and Counseling, 98,* 1287–1289.

Devine, P. G., & Monteith, M. J. (1999). Automaticity and control in stereotyping. In S. Chaiken & Y. Trope (Eds.), *Dual-process theories in social psychology* (pp. 339–360). New York, NY: Guilford Press.

Dolev, J. C., Friedlaender, L. K., & Braverman, I. M. (2001). Use of fine art to enhance visual diagnostic skills. *Journal of the American Medical Association, 286,* 1920–1921.

Dovidio, J. F., Gaertner, S. L., Kawakami, K., & Hodson, G. (2002). Why can't we just get along? Interpersonal biases and interracial distrust. *Cultural Diversity and Ethnic Minority Psychology, 8,* 88–102.

Dovidio, J. F., Gaertner, S. L., Stewart, T. L., Esses, V. M., & ten Vergert, M. (2004). From intervention to outcomes: Processes in the reduction of bias. In W. G. Stephan & P. Vogt (Eds.), *Intergroup relations programs: Practice, research and theory* (pp. 243–265). New York: New York Teachers College Press.

Duchan, J. F. (2004). Commentary: Where is the person in the ICF? *Advances in Speech-Language Pathology, 6,* 63–65.

Duffy, A. (2009). Guiding students through reflective practice—The preceptors experience: A qualitative descriptive study. *Nurse Education in Practice, 9,* 166–175.

Easton, G. (2016). How medical teachers use narratives in lectures: A qualitative study. *BMC Medical Education, 16.* doi:10.1186/s12909-015-0498-8

Elad-Strenger, J., & Littman-Ovadia, H. (2012). The contribution of the counselor–client working alliance to career exploration. *Journal of Career Assessment, 20,* 140–153. doi:10.1177/1069072711420850

Elliott, R., Bohart, A. C., Watson, J. C., & Greenberg, L. S. (2011). Empathy. In J. C. Norcross (Ed.), *Psychotherapy relationships that work: Evidence-based responsiveness* (2nd ed., pp. 132–152). New York, NY: Oxford University Press.

Emerick, L. L., & Hatten, J. T. (1974). *Diagnosis and evaluation in speech pathology.* Englewood Cliffs, NJ: Prentice-Hall, Inc.

Engel, G. L. (1977). The need for a new medical model: A challenge for biomedicine. *Science, 196,* 129–136.

Engel, G. L. (1997). From biomedical to biopsychosocial: Being scientific in the human domain. *Psychosomatics, 38,* 521–528.

Engel, J. D., Zarconi, J., Pethtel, L. L., & Missimi, S. A. (2008). *Narrative in health care: Healing patients, practitioners, profession, and community*. New York, NY: Radcliffe.

Epstein, L. (2008). Clinical therapy data as learning process: The first year of clinical training and beyond. *Topics in Language Disorders, 28*, 274–285.

Epstein, R. M., Morse, D. S., Williams, G. C., le Roux, P., Suchman, A. L., & Quill, T. E. (2003). Clinical practice and the biopsychosocial model. In R. M. Frankel, T. E. Quill, & S. H. McDaniel (Eds.), *The biopsychosocial approach: Past, present, future* (pp. 33–66). Rochester, NY: University of Rochester Press.

Erdman, S. A. (1994). Self-assessment: From research focus to research tool. In J.-P. Gagné & N. Tye-Murray (Eds.), *Research in audiological rehabilitation: Current trends and future directions, Journal of the Academy of Rehabilitative Audiology, 27* (Monograph Suppl.), 67–90.

Erdman, S. A. (2013). The biopsychosocial approach in patient- and relationship-centered care: Implications for audiologic counseling. In J. Montano & J. Spitzer (Eds.), *Adult audiologic rehabilitation* (2nd ed., pp. 159–206). San Diego, CA: Plural Publishing.

Ericsson, K. A. (2015). Acquisition and maintenance of medical expertise: a perspective from the expert-performance approach with deliberate practice. *Academic Medicine, 90*, 1471–1486.

F'arkinson, K., & Rae, J. P. (1996). The understanding and use of counselling by speech and language therapists at different levels of experience. *European Journal of Disorders of Communication, 31*, 140–152.

Facione, N. C., Facione, P. A., Sanchez, C. A. (1994). Critical thinking disposition as a measure of competent clinical judgment: The development of the California Critical Thinking Disposition Inventory. *Journal of Nursing Education, 33*, 345–350.

Facione, P. A., Facione, N. C., & Giancarlo, C. A. (2000). *Test manual: The California Critical Thinking Dispositions Inventory*. Millbrae, CA: Insight Assessment.

Facione, P. A., Sanchez, C. A., Facione, N. C., & Gainen, J. (1995). The disposition toward critical thinking. *Journal of General Education, 44*, 1–25.

Fadiman, A. (1997). *The spirit catches you and you fall down: A Hmong child, her American doctors, and the collision of two cultures*. New York, NY: Farrar, Strauss, & Giroux.

Ferguson, A., & Armstrong, E. (2004). Reflections on speech-language therapists' talk: Implications for clinical practice and education. *International Journal of Language and Communication Disorders, 39*, 469–507.

Fine, G. H. (1996). Justifying work: Occupational resources as rhetorics in restaurant kitchens. *Administrative Sciences Quarterly, 41*, 90–115.

Finn, P. (2011). Critical thinking: Knowledge and skills for evidence-based practice. *Language, Speech, and Hearing Services in Schools, 42*, 69–72.

Finn, P., Brundage, S. B., & DiLollo, A. (2016). Preparing our future helping professionals become critical thinkers: A tutorial. *Perspectives of the ASHA Special Interest Groups* (SIG 10), *1*, 43–68.

Fiske, S. T. (2002). What we know about bias and intergroup conflict, the problem of the century. *Current Directions in Psychological Science, 11*, 123–128.

Fiske, S. T., Lin, M., & Neuberg, S. L. (1999). The continuum model: Ten years later. In S. Chaiken & Y. Trope (Eds.), *Dual process theories in social psychology* (pp. 231–254). New York, NY: Guilford Press.

Flecha, R. (1999). Modern and postmodern racism in Europe: Dialogic approach and anti-racist pedagogies. *Harvard Educational Review, 69*, 150–171.

Floyd, J., Zebrowski, P. M., & Flamme, G. A. (2007). Stages of change and stuttering: A preliminary view. *Journal of Fluency Disorders, 32*, 95–120.

Flückiger, C., Del Re, A. C., Wampold, B. E., Symonds, D., & Horvath, A. O. (2012). How central is the alliance in psychotherapy? A multilevel longitudinal meta-analysis. *Journal of Counseling Psychology, 59*, 10–17.

Fourie, R. J. (2009). Qualitative study of the therapeutic relationship in speech and language therapy: Perspectives of adults with acquired communication and swallowing disorders. *International Journal of Language and Communication Disorders, 44*, 979–999.

Fourie, R. J., Crowley, N., & Oliviera, A. (2011). A qualitative exploration of therapeutic relationships from the perspective of six children receiving speech-language therapy. *Topics in Language Disorders, 31*, 310–324.

Fred, H. L. (2014). Editorial commentary. *Texas Heart Institute Journal, 41*, 251.

Friedberg, M. W., Chen, P. G., Van Busum, K. R., Aunon, F. M., Pham, C., Caloveras, J. P., . . . , Tutty, M. (2013). *Factors affecting physician professional satisfaction and their implications for patient care, health systems, and health policy.* Santa Monica, CA: RAND Corporation.

Friel-Patti, S., DesBarres, K., & Thibodeau, L. (2001). Case studies of children using Fast ForWord. *American Journal of Speech-Language Pathology, 10*, 203–215.

Gaertner, S. L., & Dovidio, J. F. (2000). *Reducing intergroup bias: The common ingroup identity model.* Philadelphia, PA: U.S. Psychology Press.

Gagné, J-P., Jennings, M. B., & Southall, K. (2013). The international classification of functioning: Implications and applications to audiologic rehabilitation. In J. Montano & J. Spitzer (Eds.), *Adult audiologic rehabilitation* (2nd ed., pp. 35–55). San Diego, CA: Plural Publishing.

Gallagher, L., Lawler, D., Brady, V., OBoyle, C., Deasy, A., & Muldoon, K. (2017). An evaluation of the appropriateness and effectiveness of structured reflection for midwifery students in Ireland. *Nurse Education in Practice, 22*, 7–14.

Geller, E., & Foley, G. M. (2009). Expanding the "ports of entry" for speech-language pathologists: A relational and reflective model for clinical practice. *American Journal of Speech-Language Pathology, 18*, 4–21.

Geller, G., Faden, R. R., & Levine, D. M. (1990). Tolerance for ambiguity among medical students: Implications for their selection, training and practice. *Social Science & Medicine, 31*, 619–624.

Gerlach, H., & Subramanian, A. (2016). Qualitative analysis of bibliotherapy as a tool for adults who stutter and graduate students. *Journal of Fluency Disorders, 47*, 1–12.

Gillam, R. B., Loeb, D. F., Hoffman, L. M., Bohman, T., Champlin, C. A., Thibodeau, L., . . . , Friel-Patti, S. (2008). The efficacy of Fast ForWord language intervention in school-age children with language impairment: A randomized controlled trial. *Journal of Speech, Language, and Hearing Research, 51*, 97–119.

Gillespie-Lynch, K., Sepeta, L., Wang, Y., Marshall, S., Gomez, L., Sigman, M., & Hutman, T. (2012). Early childhood predictors of the social competence of adults with autism. *Journal of Autism and Developmental Disorders, 42*, 161–174.

Godsey, S. R. (2011). Student perceptions of professional identity and cultural competence. (Doctoral dissertation). ProQuest Information & Learning. (3457068)

Goldberg, S. A. (1997). *Clinical skills for speech-language pathologists.* Clifton Park, NY: Delmar Cengage Learning.

Goldie, J. (2012). The formation of professional identity in medical students: Considerations for educators. *Medical Teacher, 34,* e641–e648. doi:10.3109/0142159X .2012.687476

Grais, I. M. (2014). Born to observe. *Texas Heart Institute Journal, 41,* 250–251.

Grawburg, M., Howe, T., Worrall, L., & Scarinci, N. (2013). Describing the impact of aphasia on close family members using the ICF framework. *Disability Rehabilitation, 36,* 1184–1195.

Grenness, C., Hickson, L., Laplante-Lévesque, A., & Davidson, B. (2014). Patient-centred audiological rehabilitation: Perspectives of older adults who own hearing aids. *International Journal of Audiology, 53,* S68–S75.

Grenness, C., Hickson, L., Laplante-Lévesque, A., Meyer, C., & Davidson, B. (2015a). Communication patterns in audiologic rehabilitation history-taking: Audiologists, patients, and their companions. *Ear and Hearing, 36,* 191–204.

Grenness, C., Hickson, L., Laplante-Lévesque, A., Meyer, C., & Davidson, B. (2015b). The nature of communication throughout diagnosis and management planning in initial audiologic rehabilitation consultations. *Journal of the American Academy of Audiology, 26,* 36–60.

Gwyer, J. (1999). Expert practice in pediatrics: When work is play. In G. M. Jensen, J. Gwyer, L. M. Hack, & K. F. Shepard (Eds.), *Expertise in physical therapy practice* (pp. 77–103). Boston, MA: Butterworth Heinemann.

Habl, S., Mintz, D. L., & Bailey, A. (2010). The role of therapy in psychiatric residency training: A survey of psychiatry training directors. *Academic Psychiatry, 34,* 21–26.

Hall, D. T. (1987). Careers and socialization. *Journal of Management, 13,* 301–322.

Hall, N. E. (2016). Teaching observation skills: A survey of CSD program practices. *Contemporary Issues in Communication Science and Disorders, 43,* 98–105.

Halstead, L. S. (2001). The power of compassion and caring in rehabilitation healing. *Archives of Physical Medicine and Rehabilitation, 82,* 149–154.

Hambrecht, G., & Rice, T. (2011). *Clinical observation: A guide for students in speech, language and hearing.* Sudbury, MA: Jones & Bartlett Learning.

Hardin, R. M., & Gleeson, F. A. (1979). Assessment of clinical competence using an objective structured clinical examination (OSCE). *Medical Education, 13,* 41–51.

Haron, Y., & Tran, D. (2014). Patients' perceptions of what makes a good doctor and nurse in an Israeli mental health hospital. *Issues in Mental Health Nursing, 35,* 672–679.

Haynes, W. O., & Oratio, A. R. (1978). A study of clients' perceptions of therapeutic effectiveness. *Journal of Speech and Hearing Disorders, 43,* 21–33.

Hewstone, M., Rubin, M., & Willis, H. (2002). Intergroup bias. *Annual Review of Psychology, 53,* 575–604.

Higgs, J., & McAllister, L. (2007). Educating clinical educators: Using the model of the experience of being a clinical educator. *Medical Teacher, 29,* e51–e57.

Hill, A. E., Davidson, B. J., & Theodoros, D. G. (2012). Reflections on clinical learning in novice speech-language therapy students. *International Journal of Language and Communication Disorders, 47,* 413–426.

Hojat, M., Vergare, M. J., Maxwell, K., Brainard, G., Herrine, S. K., Isenbergm, G. A., . . . , Gonnella, J. S. (2009). The devil is in the third year: A longitudinal study of erosion of empathy in medical school. *Academic Medicine, 84,* 1182–1191.

Hooper, C. R. (1996). Forming a therapeutic alliance with older adults. *ASHA, 38,* 43–45.

Horton, S., Bing, S., Bunning, K., & Pring, T. (2004). Teaching and learning speech and language therapy skills: The effectiveness of classroom as clinic in speech and language therapy student education. *International Journal of Language and Communication Disorders, 39,* 365–390.

Horvath, A., Del Re, A. C., Flückiger, C., & Symonds, D. (2011). Alliance in individual psychotherapy. *Psychotherapy, 48,* 9–16. doi:10.1037/a0022186

Howe, T. J. (2008). The ICF contextual factors related to speech-language pathology. *International Journal of Speech-Language Pathology, 10,* 27–37.

Howells, S., Barton, G., & Westerveld, M. (2016). Exploring the development of cultural awareness amongst post-graduate speech-language pathology students. *International Journal of Speech-Language Pathology, 18,* 259–271.

Husserl, E. (1970). *The idea of phenomenology.* The Hague, the Netherlands: Nijhoff.

Huth, E. J., & Murray, T. J. (Eds.) (2006). *Medicine in quotations: Views of health and disease through the ages.* Philadelphia, PA: American College of Physicians.

Ibarra, H. (1999). Provisional selves: Experimenting with image and identity in professional adaptations. *Administrative Science Quarterly, 44,* 764–791.

Jaarsma, T., Jarodzka, H., Nap, M., van Merriënboer, J. J. G., & Boshuizen, H. P. A. (2015). Expertise in clinical pathology: Combining the visual and cognitive perspective. *Advances in Health Science Education, 20,* 1089–1106.

Jacobs, S. (2016). Reflective learning, reflective practice. *Nursing, 46,* 62–64.

Jarvis-Selinger, S., Pratt, D. D., & Regehr, G. (2012). Competence isn't enough: Integrating identity formation into the medical education discourse. *Academic Medicine, 87,* 1185–1191.

Jennings, L., D'Rozario, V., Goh, M., Sovereign, A., Brogger, M., & Skovholt, T. (2008). Psychotherapy expertise in Singapore: A qualitative investigation. *Psychotherapy Research, 18,* 508–522.

Jennings, L., Goh, M., Skovholt, T. M., Hanson, M., & Banerjee-Stevens, D. (2003). Multiple factors in the development of the expert counselor and therapist. *Journal of Career Development, 30,* 59–72.

Jennings, L., Hanson, M., Skovholt, T. M., & Grier, T. (2005). Searching for mastery. *Journal of Mental Health Counseling, 27,* 19–31.

Johnson, A., Prelock, P., & Apel, K. (2016). IPE 101: Introduction to interprofessional education and practice for speech-language pathology. In A. Johnson (Ed.), *Interprofessional education and interprofessional practice in communication sciences and disorders: An introduction and case-based examples of implementation in education and health care settings* (pp. 1–28). Rockville, MD: American Speech-Language-Hearing Association.

Johnson, R. L., Saha, S., Arboleaz, J. J., Beach, M. C., & Cooper, L. A. (2004). Racial and ethnic differences in patient perceptions of bias and cultural competence in health care. *Journal of General and Internal Medicine, 19,* 101–110.

Justice, L. M., Jiang, H., Logan, J. A., & Schmitt, M. B. (2017). Predictors of language gains among school-age children with language impairment in the public schools. *Journal of Speech, Language and Hearing Research, 60,* 1–16. doi:10.1044/2016 _JSLHR-L-16-0026. Retrieved May 26, 2017.

Katz, J. T., & Khoshbin, S. (2014). Can visual arts training improve physician performance? *Transactions of the American Clinical and Climatological Association, 125,* 331–341.

Kawakami, K., Dovidio, J. F., Moll, J., Hermsen, S., & Russin, A. (2000). Just say no (to stereotyping): Effects of training in the negation of stereotypic associations on stereotype activation. *Journal of Personality and Social Psychology, 78*, 871–888.

Kay-Raining Bird, E., & Eriks-Brophy, A. (2011). From the guest editors. Introduction to the special issue of service delivery to First Nations, Inuit and Métis in Canada: Part 1. *Canadian Journal of Speech-Language Pathology and Audiology, 35*, 106–107.

Kazdin, A. E. (2003). Assessment and evaluation of interventions. In A. E. Kazdin (Ed.), *Research design in clinical psychology* (pp. 408–435). Needham Heights, MA: Allyn & Bacon.

King, G., Currie, M., Bartlett, D. J., Gilpin, M., Willoughby, C., Tucker, M. A., . . . , Baxter, D. (2007). The development of expertise in pediatric rehabilitation therapists: Changes in approach, self-knowledge, and use of enabling and customizing strategies. *Developmental Neurorehabilitation, 10*, 223–240.

King, G., Currie, M., Bartlett, D. J., Strachan, D., Tucker, M. A., & Willoughby, C. (2008). The development of expertise in paediatric rehabilitation therapists: The roles of motivation, openness to experience, and types of caseload experience. *Australian Occupational Therapy Journal, 55*, 108–122.

Kirkman, M. A. (2013). Deliberate practice, domain-specific expertise, and implications for surgical education in current climes. *Journal of Surgical Education, 70*, 309–317.

Kivighlan, D. M., & Quigley, S. T. (1991). Dimensions used by experienced and novice group therapists to conceptualize group process. *Journal of Counseling Psychology, 38*, 415–423.

Klevans, D. R., Volz, H. B., & Friedman, R. M. (1981). A comparison of experiential and observational approaches for enhancing the interpersonal communication skills of speech-language pathology students. *Journal of Speech and Hearing Disorders, 46*, 208–213.

Klugman, C. M., Peel, J., & Beckman-Mendez, D. (2011). Art rounds: Teaching interprofessional students visual thinking strategies at one school. *Arts and Medical Education, 86*, 1266–1271.

Knight, L. V., & Mattick, K. (2006). 'When I first came here, I thought medicine was black and white': Making sense of medical students' ways of knowing. *Social Science and Medicine, 63*, 1084–1096.

Koh, Y. H., Wong, M. L., & Lee, J. J-M. (2014). Medical students' reflective writing about a task-based learning experience on public health communication. *Medical Teacher, 36*, 121–129.

Kröner-Herwig, B., Zachriat, C., & Weigand, D. (2006). Do patient characteristics predict outcome in the outpatient treatment of chronic tinnitus? *GMS Psycho-Social-Medicine, 3*, Doc07. Retrieved May 26, 2017 from http://www.egms.de/en/journals/psm/2006-3/psm000027.shtml

Kururi, N., Tozato, F., Lee, B., Kazama, H., Katsuyama, S., Takahashi, M., . . . , Watanabe, H. (2016). Professional identity acquisition process model in interprofessional education using structural equation modelling: A 10-year initiative survey. *Journal of Interprofessional Care, 30*, 175–183.

Lambert, M. J. (1992). Psychotherapy outcome research: Implications for integrative and eclectic therapists. In J. C. Norcross & M. R. Goldfried (Eds.), *Handbook of psychotherapy integration* (pp. 94–129). New York, NY: Basic Books.

Lambert, M. J., Smart, D. W., Campbell, M. P., Hawkins, E. J., Harmon, C., & Slade, K. L. (2006). Psychotherapy outcome as measured by the OQ-45 I African American, Asian/Pacific Islander, Latino/a, and Native American clients compared with matched Caucasian clients. *Journal of College Student Psychotherapy, 20*, 17–29.

Laplante-Lévesque, A., Hickson, L., & Grenness, C. (2014). An Australian survey of audiologists' preferences for patient-centredness. *International Journal of Audiology, 53*, S76–S82. doi: 10.3109/14992027.2013.832418

Laplante-Lévesque, A., Hickson, L., & Worrall, L. (2010). A qualitative study on shared decision making in rehabilitative audiology. *Journal of the American Academy of Audiology, 43*, 27–43.

Laska, K. M., Smith, T. L., Wislocki, A., Minami, T., & Wampold, B. E. (2013). Uniformity in evidence based treatment? Therapist effects in the delivery of cognitive processing therapy in treatment of PTSD. *Journal of Counseling Psychology, 60*, 31–41.

Law, J., Garrett, Z., & Nye, C. (2004). The efficacy of treatment for children with developmental speech and language delay/disorder: A meta-analysis. *Journal of Speech, Language, and Hearing Research, 47*, 924–943.

Lazarus, R. S., & Folkman, S. (1984). *Stress, appraisal, and coping.* New York, NY: Springer.

Lee, K., Manning, W. H., & Herder, C. (2015). Origin and pawn scaling for adults who do and do not stutter: A preliminary comparison. *Journal of Fluency Disorders, 45*, 73–81.

Leonard, D., & Swap, W. (2005). *Deep smarts: How to cultivate and transfer enduring business wisdom.* Boston, MA: Harvard Business School Press.

Lilienfeld, S. O., Marshall, J., Todd, J. T., & Shane, H. C. (2014). The persistence of fad interventions in the face of negative scientific evidence: Facilitated communication for autism as a case example. *Evidence-Based Communication Assessment and Intervention, 8*, 62–101. doi:10.1080/17489539.2014.976332

Lindquist, I., Enghardt, M., Garnham, L., Poland, F., & Richardson, B. (2006). Physiotherapy students' professional identity on the edge of working life. *Medical Teacher, 28*, 270–276.

Locke, J., Williams, J., Shih, W., & Kasari, C. (2017). Characteristics of socially successful elementary school-aged children with autism. *Journal of Child Psychology and Psychiatry, 58*, 94–102. doi: 10.1111/jcpp.12636

Looi, V., Lee, Z. Z., & Loo, J. H. Y. (2016). Quality of life outcomes for children with hearing impairment in Singapore. *International Journal of Pediatric Otorhinolaryngology, 80*, 88–100.

Lund, M. L., Tamm, M., & Bränholm, I. B. (2001). Patients' perceptions of their participation in rehabilitation planning and professionals' view of their strategies to encourage it. *Occupational Therapy International, 8*, 151–167.

Luterman, D. (2017). *Counseling persons with communication disorders and their families* (6th ed.). Austin, TX: Pro-Ed, Inc.

Lutz, G., Roling, G., Berger, B., Edelhäuser, F., & Scheffer, C. (2016). Reflective practice and its role in facilitating creative responses to dilemmas within clinical communication—A qualitative analysis. *BMC Medical Education, 16*, 301–309.

Macran, S., & Shapiro, D. A. (1998). The role of personal therapy for therapists: A review. *British Journal of Medical Psychology, 71*, 13–25.

Malikiosi-Loizos, M. (2013). Personal therapy for future therapists: Reflections on a still-debated issue. *The European Journal of Counselling Psychology, 2*, 33–50.

Mamede, S., & Schmidt, H. G. (2004). The structure of reflective practice in medicine. *Medical Education, 38*, 1302–1308.

Mann, K., Gordon, J., & MacLeod, A. (2009). Reflection and reflective practice in health professions: A systematic review. *Advances in Health Sciences Education, 12*, 549–621.

Mann, L., Howard, P., Nowens, F., & Martin, F. (2008). Professional identity: A framework for research in engineering education. *Proceedings of the 19th Annual Conference for Australasian Association for Engineering Education*. Yeppoon, Queensland, Australia.

Manning, W. H. (2010). Evidence of clinically significant change: The therapeutic alliance and the possibility of outcomes-informed care. *Seminars in Speech and Language, 31*, 207–216.

Manton, R. (2004). Are observation skills at risk? *Update, 68*, 5.

Marañón, A. A., & Pera, M. P. I. (2015). Theory and practice in the construction of professional identity in nursing students: A qualitative study. *Nursing Education Today, 35*, 859–863.

Margalit, A. P. A., & El-Ad, A. (2008). Costly patients with unexplained medical symptoms: A high-risk population. *Patient Education and Counseling, 70*, 173–178.

Margalit, A. P. A., Glick, S. M., Benbassat, J., & Cohen, A. (2004). Effect of a biopsychosocial approach on patient satisfaction and patterns of care. *Journal of General Medicine, 19*, 485–491.

Marmot, M. (2005). Social determinants of health inequalities. *Lancet, 365*, 1099–1104.

Martin, J., Slemon, A. G., Hiebert, B., Hallberg, E. T., & Cummings, A. L. (1989). Conceptualizations of novice and experienced counselors. *Journal of Counseling Psychology, 36*, 395–400.

Masdonati, J., Perdrix, S., Massoudi, K., & Rossier, J. (2014). Working alliance as a moderator and a mediator of career counseling effectiveness. *Journal of Career Assessment, 22*, 3–17. doi:10.1177/1069072713487489

McClellan, K. M., McCann, C. M., Worrall, L. E., & Harwood, M. L. N. (2014). Māori experiences of aphasia therapy: "But I'm from Hauiti and we've got shags." *International Journal of Speech-Language Pathology, 16*, 529–540.

McHugh, M. D., & Lake, E. T. (2010). Understanding clinical expertise: Nurse education, experience and the hospital context. *Research in Nursing and Health, 33*, 276–287.

McLain, D. L., Keffalonitis, E., & Armani, K. (2015). Ambiguity tolerance in organizations: Definitional clarification and perspectives on future research. *Frontiers in Psychology, 6*, 344. DOI: 10.3389/fpsyg.2015.00344

Meilijson, S., & Katzenberger, I. (2014). A clinical education program for speech-language pathologists applying reflective practice, evidence-practice and case-based learning. *Folia Phoniatrica et Logopaedica, 66*, 158–163.

Meza, J. P., & Passermann, D. S. (2011). *Integrating narrative medicine and evidence-based medicine: The everyday social practice of healing*. New York, NY: Radcliffe.

Millard, S. K., & Cook, F. M. (2010). Working with young children who stutter: Raising our game. *Seminars in Speech and Language, 31*, 250–261.

Miller, A., Grohe, M., Khoshbin, S., & Katz, J. T. (2013). From the galleries to the clinic: Applying art museum lessons to patient care. *Journal of Medical Humanities, 34*, 433–438.

Miranda, C., Veatch, P. M., Martyr, M. A., & LeRoy, B. S. (2016). Portrait of the master genetic counselor clinician: A qualitative investigation of expertise in genetic counseling. *Journal of Genetic Counseling, 25*, 767–785.

Morrison, T. L., & Smith, J. D. (2013). Working alliance development in occupational therapy: A cross case analysis. *Australian Occupational Therapy Journal, 60*, 326–333. doi:10.1111/1440-1630.12053

Mostert, M. P. (2001). Facilitated communication since 1995: A review of published studies. *Journal of Autism and Developmental Disorders, 31*, 287–313.

Multon, K. D., Ellis-Kalton, C., Heppner, M. J., & Gysbers, N. C. (2003). The relationship between counselor verbal response modes and the working alliance in career counseling. *The Career Development Quarterly, 51*, 259–273.

Naber, J., & Wyatt, T. H. (2014). The effect of reflective writing interventions on the critical thinking skills and dispositions of baccalaureate nursing students. *Nurse Education Today, 34*, 67–72.

Naghshineh, S., Hafler, J. P., Miller, A. R., Blancos, M. A., Lipsitz, S. R., Dubroff, R. P., . . . , Katz, J. T. (2008). Formal art observation improves medical students' visual diagnostic skills. *Journal of General Internal Medicine, 23*, 991–997.

Nahmias, A. S., Kase, C., & Mandell, D. S. (2014). Comparing cognitive outcomes among children with autism spectrum disorders receiving community-based early intervention in one of three placements. *Autism: The International Journal of Research and Practice, 18*, 311–320.

Newton, B. W., Barber, L., Clardy, J., Cleveland, E., & O'Sullivan, P. (2008). Is there hardening of the heart during medical school? *Academic Medicine: Journal of the Association of American Medical Colleges, 83*, 244–249.

Nicholson, N. (1984). A theory of work role transitions. *Administrative Science Quarterly, 29*, 172–191.

Novak, D. H., Epstein, R. M., & Paulsen, R. H. (1999). Toward creating physician-healers: Fostering medical students' self-awareness, personal growth and well-being. *Academic Medicine, 74*, 516–520.

O'Halloran, R., & Larkins, B. (2008). The ICF activities and participation as related to speech-language pathology. *International Journal of Speech-Language Pathology, 10*, 18–26.

Öberg, M., Lunner, T., & Andersson, G. (2007). Psychometric evaluation of hearing specific self-report measures and their associations with psychosocial and demographic variables. *Audiological Medicine, 5*, 188–199.

Oelke, N. D., Thurson, W. E., & Arthur, N. (2013). Intersections between interprofessional practice, cultural competency, and primary healthcare. *Journal of Interprofessional Care, 27*, 367–372.

Oratio, A. R. (1976). A factor-analytic study of criteria for evaluating student clinicians in speech pathology. *Journal of Communication Disorders, 9*, 99–110.

Oratio, A. R. (1980). Dimensions of therapeutic behavior. *Journal of Communication Disorders, 13*, 213–230.

Oratio, A. R., & Hood, S. B. (1977). Certain select variables as predictors of goal achievement in speech therapy. *Journal of Communication Disorders, 10*, 331–342.

Orlinsky, D., Rønnestad, M. H., Ambühl, H., Willutzki, U., Botermans, J.-F., Cierpka, M., . . . , Davis, M. (1999). Psychotherapists' assessment of their development at different career levels. *Psychotherapy, 36*, 203–215.

Orlinsky, D., Rønnestad, M. H., & Willutzki, U. (2004). Fifty years of psychotherapy process-outcome research: Continuity and change. In D. J. Lambert (Ed.), *Bergin and Garfield's handbook of psychotherapy and behavior change* (5th ed., pp. 307–390). Hoboken, NJ: Wiley.

Otsuka, S., Uono, S., Yoshimura, S., Zhao, S., & Toichi, M. (2017). Emotion perception mediates the predictive relationship between verbal ability and functional outcome in high-functioning adults with autism spectrum disorder. *Journal of Autism and Developmental Disorders, 47*, 1166–1182. doi:10.1007/s10803-017-3036-1

Palmadottir, G. (2006). Client–therapist relationships: Experiences of occupational therapy clients in rehabilitation. *British Journal of Occupational Therapy, 69*, 394–401.

Papp, K. K., Huang, G. C., Lauzon Clabo, L. M., Delva, D., Fischer, M., Konopasek, L., . . . , Gusic, M. (2014). Milestones of critical thinking: A developmental model for medicine and nursing. *Academic Medicine, 89*, 715–720.

Pellat, G. C. (2004). Patient-professional partnership in spinal cord injury rehabilitation. *British Journal of Nursing, 13*, 948–953.

Pellechia, M., Connell, J. E., Kerns, C. M., Xie, M., Marcus, S. C., & Mandell, D. S. (2016). Child characteristics associated with outcome for children with autism in a school-based behavioral intervention. *Autism: The International Journal of Research and Practice, 20*, 321–329.

Perry, M., Maffulli, N., Wilson, S., & Morrisey, D. (2011). The effectiveness of arts-based interventions in medical education: A literature review. *Medical Education, 45*, 141–148.

Peterkin, A. D. (2016). Portfolio to go: 1000+ reflective writing prompts and provocations for clinical learners. Toronto, Ontario, Canada: University of Toronto Press.

Petersen, D. B., Gillam, S. L., Spencer, T., & Gillam, R. B. (2010). The effects of literate narrative intervention on children with neurologically based language impairments: An early stage study. *Journal of Speech, Language, and Hearing Research, 53*, 961–981.

Pickering, M. (2003). Shared territories: An element of culturally sensitive practice. *Folia Phoniatrica et Logopaedica, 55*, 287–292.

Plant, E., & Devine, P. G. (2003). The antecedents and implications of interracial anxiety. *Perspectives in Social Psychology Bulletin, 29*, 790–801.

Platzer, H., Blake, D., & Ashford, D. (2000). Barriers to learning from reflection: A study of the use of group work with post-registration nurses. *Journal of Advanced Nursing, 31*, 1001–1008.

Plexico, L. W., Manning, W. H., & DiLollo, A. (2010). Client perceptions of effective and ineffective therapeutic alliances during treatment of stuttering. *Journal of Fluency Disorders, 35*, 333–354.

Plexico, L. W., Manning, W. H., & Levitt, H. (2009). Coping responses by adults who stutter: Part I. Protecting the self and others. *Journal of Fluency Disorders, 34*, 87–107.

Poost-Foroosh, L., Jennings, M. B., & Cheesman, M. F. (2015). Comparison of client and clinician views of the importance of factors in client-clinician interaction in hearing aid purchase decisions. *Journal of the American Academy of Audiology, 26*, 247–259.

Prochaska, J. O., & DiClemente, C. C. (1984). *The transtheoretical approach: Crossing traditional boundaries of therapy*. Homewood, IL: Dow Jones-Irwin.

Rachakonda, T., Jeffe, D. B., Shin, J. J., Mankarious, L., Fanning, R. J., Lesperance, M. M., & Lieu, J. E. C. (2014). Validity, discriminative ability, and reliability of the hearing-related quality of life questionnaire for adolescents. *Laryngoscope, 124*, 570–578.

Raimy, V. C. (Ed.). (1950). *Training in clinical psychology*. New York, NY: Prentice-Hall.

Resnik, L., & Jensen, G. M. (2003). Using clinical outcomes to explore the theory of expert practice in physical therapy. *Physical Therapy, 83*, 1090–1106.

Rhodes, M. (1961). An analysis of creativity. *Phi Delta Kappa, 42*, 306–307.

Roberts, R. M., Sands, F., Gannoni, A., & Marciano, T. (2015). Perceptions of the support that mothers and fathers of children with cochlear implants received in South Australia: A qualitative study. *International Journal of Audiology, 54*, 942–950.

Rogers, C. (1957). The necessary and sufficient conditions of therapeutic change. *Journal of Consulting Psychology, 21,* 95–105.

Schattner, A., Rudin, D., & Jellin, N. (2004). Good physicians from the perspective of their patients. *BMC Health Services Research, 4*, 26–30. doi:10.1186/1472-6963-4-26.

Schaub-de Jong, M. A., & van der Schans, C. P. (2010). Teaching reflection: Speech and language therapy using visual clues for reflection. *Education for Health, 23*, 285. http://www.educationforhealth.net, IP: 130.111.46.54

Schaub-de Jong, M. A., Schönrock-Adema, J., Dekker, H., Verkerk, M., & Cohen-Schotanus, J. (2011). Development of a student rating scale to evaluate teachers' competencies for facilitating reflective learning. *Medical Education, 45*, 155–165.

Schein, E. H. (1978). *Career dynamics: Matching individual and organizational needs*. Reading, MA: Addison-Wesley.

Schlosser, R. W., Balandin, S., Hemsley, B., Iacono, T., Probst, P., & von Tetzchner, S. (2014). Facilitated communication and authorship: A systematic review. *Augmentative and Alternative Communication, 30*, 359–368. doi:10.3109/07434618.2014.971490

Shane, H. C., & Kearns, K. (1994). An examination of the role of the facilitator in "facilitated communication." *American Journal of Speech-Language Pathology, 3,* 48–54.

Shirk, S. R., & Karver, M. (2003). Prediction of treatment outcome from relationship variables in child and adolescent therapy: A meta-analytic review. *Journal of Consulting and Clinical Psychology, 71*, 452–464.

Simmons-Mackie, N., & Schultz, M. (2003). The role of humour in aphasia therapy. *Aphasia, 17*, 751–766.

Sklar, D. P. (2015). How do I figure out what I want to do if I don't know who I am supposed to be? *Academic Medicine, 90*, 695–696.

Skovholt, T. M. (2005). The cycle of caring: A model of expertise in the helping professions. *Journal of Mental Health Counseling, 27*, 82–93.

Skovholt, T. M., & Jennings, L. (2004). *Master therapists: Exploring expertise in therapy and counseling*. Boston, MA: Allyn & Bacon.

Skovholt, T. M., & Jennings, L. (2005). Mastery and expertise in counseling. *Journal of Mental Health Counseling, 27*, 13–18.

Skovholt, T. M., Jennings, L., & Mullenbach, M. (2004). Portrait of the master therapist: Developmental model of the highly functioning self. In T. M. Skovholt & L. Jennings (Eds.), *Master therapists: Exploring expertise in therapy and counseling* (pp. 125–146). Boston, MA: Allyn & Bacon.

Slay, H. S., & Smith, D. A. (2011). Personal identity construction: Using narrative to understand the negotiation of professional and stigmatized cultural identities. *Human Relations, 64*, 85–107.

Sobral, D. T. (2000). An appraisal of medical students' reflection-in-learning. *Medical Education, 34*, 182–187.

Sobral, D. T. (2005). Medical students' mindset for reflective learning: A revalidation study of the reflection-in-learning scale. *Advances in Health Sciences Education, 10*, 303–310.

Soler, J. K., & Okkes, I. (2012). Reasons for encounter and symptom diagnoses: A superior description of patients' problems in contrast to medically unexplained symptoms (MUS). *Family Practice, 29*, 272.

Stech, E. L., Curtiss, J. W., Troesch, P. J., & Binnie, C. (1973). Clients reinforcement of speech clinicians: A factor-analytic study. *Asha 15*:287–289.

Stein, D. M., & Lambert, M. J. (1995). Graduate training in psychotherapy: Are therapy outcomes enhanced? *Journal of Consulting and Clinical Psychology, 63*, 182–196.

Steinhausen, H.-C., Mohr Jensen, C., & Lauritsen, M. B. (2016). A systematic review and meta-analysis of the long-term overall outcome of autism spectrum disorders in adolescence and adulthood. *Acta Psychiatrica Scandinavica, 133*, 445–452. doi:10.1111/acps.12559

Stricker, G. (2002). What is a scientist-practitioner anyway? *Journal of Clinical Psychology, 58*, 1277–1283. doi:10.1002/jclp.10111

Theodoroff, S. M., Schuette, A., Griest, S., & Henry, J. A. (2014). Individual patient factors associated with effective tinnitus treatment. *Journal of the American Academy of Audiology, 25*, 631–643.

Thistlethwaite, J. (2016). Interprofessional education: 50 years and counting. *Medical Education, 50*, 1082–1086.

Thistlethwaite, J., & Moran, M. (2010). Learning outcomes for interprofessional education (IPE): Literature review and synthesis. *Journal of Interprofessional Care, 23*, 501–513.

Thompson, L., & McCabe, R. (2015). The effect of clinician-patient alliance and communication on treatment adherence in mental health care: A systematic review. *Psychiatry, 12*, 87. doi:10.1037/t05559-000

Threats, T. T. (2010). The ICF and speech-language pathology: Aspiring to a fuller realization of ethical and moral issues. *International Journal of Speech-Language Pathology, 12*, 87–93.

Tickle-Degnen, L. (2002). Client-centered practice, therapeutic relationship, and the use of research evidence. *The American Journal of Occupational Therapy, 56*, 471–474.

Tickle-Degnen, L., & Gavett, E. (2003). Changes in nonverbal behavior during the development of therapeutic relationships. In P. Philippot, E. J. Coats, & R. S. Feldman (Eds.), *Nonverbal behavior in clinical settings* (pp. 75–110). New York, NY: Oxford University Press.

Tonge, B. J., & Einfeld, S. L. (2003). Psychopathology and intellectual disability: The Australian child to adult longitudinal study. In L. M. Glidden (ed.), *International review of research in mental retardation* (Vol. 26, pp. 61–91). New York, NY: Academic Press.

Tostanoski, A., Lang, R., Raulston, T., Carnett, A., & Davis, T. (2014). Voices from the past: Comparing the rapid prompting method and facilitated communication.

Developmental Neurorehabilitation, 17(4), 219–223. doi:10.3109/17518423.2012.749952

Travers, J. C., Tincani, M. J., & Lang, R. (2014). Facilitated communication denies people with disabilities their voice. *Research and Practice for Persons with Severe Disabilities, 39(3),* 195–202. doi:10.1177/1540796914556778

Ulvenes, P. G., Berggraf, L., Hoffart, A., Stiles, T. C., Svartberg, M., McCullough, L., & Wampold, B. E. (2012). Different processes for different therapies: Therapist actions, therapeutic bond, and outcome. *Psychotherapy, 49,* 291–302.

Volz, H. B., Klevans, D. R., Norton, S. J., & Putens, D. L. (1978). Interpersonal communication skills of speech-language pathology undergraduates: The effects of training. *Journal of Speech and Hearing Disorders, 43,* 524–542.

Votruba, K. L., Rapport, L. J., Whitman, R. D., Johnson, A., & Langenecker, S. (2013). Personality differences among patients with chronic aphasia predict improvement in speech-language therapy. *Topics in Stroke Rehabilitation, 20,* 421–431.

Wade, C., Tavris, C., & Garry, M. (2014). *Psychology* (11th ed.). Upper Saddle River, NJ: Prentice Hall.

Wald, H. S. (2015). Personal identity (trans)formation in medical education: Reflection, relationship, resilience. *Academic Medicine, 90,* 701–706.

Wald, H. S., Anthony, D., Hutchinson, T. A., Liben, S., Smilovitch, M., & Donato, A. (2015). Professional identity formation in medical education for humanistic, resilient physicians: Pedagogic strategies for bridging theory to practice. *Academic Medicine, 90,* 753–760.

Walker, S. E. (2003). Active learning strategies to promote critical thinking. *Journal of Athletic Training, 38,* 263–267.

Wampold, B. E. (2001). *The great psychotherapy debate: Models, methods, and findings.* Mahwah, NJ: Erlbaum.

Warmington, S., & McColl, G. (2016). Medical student stories of participation in patient-related activities: The construction of relational identity. *Advances in Health Sciences Education.* doi:10.1007/s10459-016-9689-2

Washington, K. N., Thomas-Stonell, N., McLeod, S., & Warr-Leeper, G. (2015). Outcomes and predictors in preschoolers with speech-language and/or developmental mobility impairments. *Child Language Teaching and Therapy, 31,* 141–157.

Wayne, S., Delmore, D., Serna, L., Jerabek, R., Timm, C., & Kalishman, S. (2011). The association between intolerance for ambiguity and decline in medical students' attitudes toward the underserved. *Academic Medicine, 86,* 877–882.

Wellbery, C., & McAteer, R. A. (2015). The art of observation: A pedagogical framework. *Academic Medicine, 90,* 1624–1630.

Wells, M. I. (2000). Beyond cultural competence: A model for individual and institutional cultural development. *Journal of Community Health Nursing, 17,* 189–199.

Whiston, S. C., Rossier, J., & Hernandez Barón, P. M. (2016). The working alliance in career counseling: A systematic overview. *Journal of Career Assessment, 24,* 591–604.

White, A. A. (2011). *Seeing patients: Unconscious bias in health care.* Cambridge, MA: Harvard University Press.

White, S., Ollendick, T., & Bray, B. (2011). College students on the autism spectrum: Prevalence and associated problems. *Autism, 15,* 683–701.

Wilkinson, R., & Marmot, M. (2003). *The solid facts* (2nd ed.). Copenhagen, Denmark: World Health Organization.

Wilson, T. D., Lindsey, S., Schooler, T. Y. (2000). A model of dual attitudes. *Psychological Review, 107,* 101–126.

World Health Organization. (1990). *International statistical classification of diseases and related health problems, Revision 10.* Geneva, Switzerland: Author.

World Health Organization. (2001). *International classification of functioning, disability and health.* Geneva, Switzerland: Author.

World Health Organization. (2007). *International classification of functioning, disability and health—Children and youth version.* Geneva, Switzerland: Author.

World Health Organization. (2011). *World health report on disability.* Geneva, Switzerland: Author.

Zraick, R. I., Allen, R. M., & Johnson, S. B. (2003). The use of standardized patients to teach and test interpersonal and communication skills with students in speech-language pathology. *Advanced in Health Sciences, 8,* 237–248.

INDEX